"Guess."

"I'm not that foolish."

"Go on," she insisted. "Guess."

How old was Sorcha?

She'd told him that she'd worked in an office before training as a nurse... Everything pointed toward mid to late twenties, but now he looked for visual clues.

Really looked.

She wore no makeup. Her lips were full and parted to reveal a white, slightly toothy smile that endeared. The blaze of wild red curls that had first caught his eye had since been tied up, but stray curls danced a little around her full cheeks and the low evening sun brought out the coppers and gold...

Beautiful.

Rather than saying that, Richard chose a far more sensible response. "Twenty-four."

'I"m guessing you took a couple of years off to be safe?"

He smiled at her perception. "Twenty-six, then?"

Those curls resumed their wayward dance as shook her head. "I'm twenty-eight." She took a sip of her wine. "What about you?"

"Guess," Richard responded, when usually he didn't play such silly games.

It was Sorcha's turn now...

Dear Reader,

Life is often unpredictable, and nowhere personifies that more than in the Accident and Emergency Department. At London's Primary Hospital the staff are used to helping patients navigate those difficult days, as well as looking out for each other.

Richard, my hero, is very English with a stiff upper lip—he knows more than most how quickly circumstances can change and has been going through a lot of late, though he prefers not to discuss personal matters. Sorcha, my gorgeous Scottish heroine, loves to talk, at least about the little things. She's flighty and funny, but beneath all that Sorcha is hiding a heart that was broken at birth.

Life is indeed unpredictable.

I decided it was time for both Sorcha and Richard to discover the other side of the coin—how an unexpected turn of events can also usher in something rather wonderful...

Happy reading,

Carol xxx

NURSE'S NINE-MONTH SURPRISE

CAROL MARINELLI

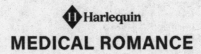

MEDICAL ROMANCE

If you purchased this book without a cover you should be aware that this book is stolen property. It was reported as "unsold and destroyed" to the publisher, and neither the author nor the publisher has received any payment for this "stripped book."

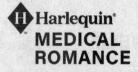

ISBN-13: 978-1-335-94304-0

Nurse's Nine-Month Surprise

Copyright © 2025 by Carol Marinelli

All rights reserved. No part of this book may be used or reproduced in any manner whatsoever without written permission.

Without limiting the author's and publisher's exclusive rights, any unauthorized use of this publication to train generative artificial intelligence (AI) technologies is expressly prohibited.

This is a work of fiction. Names, characters, places and incidents are either the product of the author's imagination or are used fictitiously. Any resemblance to actual persons, living or dead, businesses, companies, events or locales is entirely coincidental.

For questions and comments about the quality of this book, please contact us at CustomerService@Harlequin.com.

TM and ® are trademarks of Harlequin Enterprises ULC.

 Harlequin Enterprises ULC
22 Adelaide St. West, 41st Floor
Toronto, Ontario M5H 4E3, Canada
www.Harlequin.com

Printed in U.S.A.

Carol Marinelli recently filled in a form asking for her job title. Thrilled to be able to put down her answer, she put "writer." Then it asked what Carol did for relaxation and she put down the truth—"writing." The third question asked for her hobbies. Well, not wanting to look obsessed, she crossed her fingers and answered "swimming"—but, given that the chlorine in the pool does terrible things to her highlights, I'm sure you can guess the real answer!

Books by Carol Marinelli

Harlequin Medical Romance

The Nurse's Reunion Wish
Unlocking the Doctor's Secrets
The Nurse's Pregnancy Wish
One Month to Tame the Surgeon

Harlequin Presents

Heirs to the Romero Empire

His Innocent for One Spanish Night
Midnight Surrender to the Spaniard
Virgin's Stolen Nights with the Boss

Rival Italian Brothers

Italian's Pregnant Mistress
Italian's Cinderella Temptation

Wed into a Billionaire's World

Bride Under Contract
She Will Be Queen

Visit the Author Profile page at Harlequin.com for more titles.

**Praise for
Carol Marinelli**

"I really get sucked into this author's medical romances! She has a unique writing style that can be almost breathless at times."
—*Goodreads* on *The Midwife's One-Night Fling*

CHAPTER ONE

An Indian summer in London

HIS INTENTION HAD been to slip away quietly.

Dr Richard Lewis had hoped to be on the late-afternoon train or at least outside the hotel before his absence was noted. Then, when the inevitable texts arrived, asking where he was, he could fire back a one-word answer—Cardiff. Or perhaps a quick line stating that he'd be back on board tomorrow.

It was not to be.

'Richard!'

Unseen, he briefly closed his eyes in mild frustration before turning to see that both Monica and George were making their way across the hotel foyer towards him.

A large medical conference was being held in central London and they were all staying at a hotel here, near Kings Cross. There was a group of eight or so of them who had been side by side at medical school and had remained both colleagues and friends over the years.

Two of them were bearing down on him now.

Monica was now a consultant obstetrician at The Primary, in north London, and was also a speaker at the conference. George, a consultant paediatrician, also at The Primary, had just given a major presentation. Richard was neither speaking nor presenting; he was attending the conference to keep updated, as well as to get his professional development hours up.

His own once soaring career had somewhat stalled, and he currently worked as a locum accident and emergency registrar across several hospitals in London.

'We've been looking for you,' Monica said as they caught up with him. 'We're all meeting at the rooftop bar for drinks...'

'Rafi and Thomas are coming,' George added. 'Though we haven't decided where to go for dinner. Any preferences?'

'Don't make plans around me.' Richard shook his head. 'I'm not going to be here for dinner.'

'You're leaving?' Monica checked, her shoulders drooping, making no attempt to hide her disappointment. 'But I thought you were here for the entire conference?'

'I am,' Richard confirmed. 'I just can't make dinner tonight. I'll be back first thing tomorrow.'

'But we've hardly seen you since the conference started.'

'I've been at every session,' Richard pointed out. 'And I was at the dinner last night...'

'That was a formal function, though,' Monica said. 'And you were late for that—wasn't he, George?'

George flushed a little before responding, 'He wasn't *that* late.'

Richard smothered a smile. He had, in fact, been at the hotel since yesterday morning, helping his old friend prepare for his presentation, though of course George didn't want the uber-efficient Monica to know that!

George fumbled on, trying to persuade him to join them. 'A good night out with the old mob might be just the ticket...'

'It'll be like old times,' Monica urged.

It could never be like old times.

They kept on waiting for the old Richard to come back. For the man he'd been fifteen, ten, five or even three years ago to return. But that version of himself no longer existed.

Richard didn't blame them for not getting it— no doubt he looked much the same. He'd always been the tallest in their group, and at thirty-five his dark brown hair was still neat and regularly trimmed, and he was clean shaven.

Polite and measured, Richard certainly wasn't

a rule-breaker. He was predictable...possibly even a bit boring at times—though those traits had been appreciated in their salad days! And he'd always dressed well. Today proved no exception—he wore a smart navy suit, a white shirt with the top button done up, and there was a pop of colour provided by a periwinkle silk tie. Even after five p.m. it remained immaculately knotted.

Typical Richard.

Not quite.

'We'll go out tomorrow night,' Richard promised. 'We could maybe try the hotel restaurant—Spanish-Mexican... I've heard good things.'

George clearly wasn't keen, though he made it about the restaurant rather than admit it wasn't for him. 'I doubt we'd get a booking for all of us.'

'How about Indian, then?' Monica smiled at Richard. 'That's always been your favourite.'

'Sure.' Richard nodded, even though he wasn't sure if Indian was his favourite any more. 'Sounds great.'

As Monica headed for the bar George remained.

'Thanks for not saying anything about yesterday. It was good to have a trial run...'

Despite George's brilliance, he was dreadful when talking in front of an audience and had asked for Richard's help. Yesterday, without the others knowing, they had been locked away in

George's suite, ordering room service and going over and over his presentation.

'It more than paid off,' Richard said. 'You did a terrific job.'

'I'm surprised you didn't nod off. You must have heard it twenty times yesterday.'

'I learnt a lot.' Richard meant it. 'I was more than happy to help.'

'Well, it was much appreciated.' George nodded. 'And likewise, if you do ever decide to resume your studies...' George hesitated and swallowed a little awkwardly. 'I'm not trying to push, or anything. I know the others can be a bit much at times...'

Richard chose not to reveal that he was looking to sit the final exam for his Fellowship of the Royal College of Emergency Medicine in May. The decision still felt a little too new to be discussed and debated over dinner, as it inevitably would be.

'They mean well,' Richard settled for saying instead. 'I know that.' He lightly closed the conversation by glancing at his watch. 'George, much as I'd like to stay and chat, I don't want to miss my train.'

'Of course.'

This time he made it as far as the brass revolving door...

'Richard!'

Mr Field, his old boss and mentor, emerged. 'On your way out?' he checked. 'I'd advise against it.' Mr Field was very red in the face and dripping with sweat. 'It's like a damn oven out there…'

'So I've heard.' It was the last week in September, so technically autumn, but England was wilting under a heatwave. 'I believe there are a few colleagues from The Primary up at the rooftop bar if you want to make the most of the unseasonable weather.'

'I'll stay down here with the air-conditioning, thanks,' Mr Field said, and then looked Richard up and down. 'Have you lost weight or grown taller?'

'Taller,' Richard responded good-naturedly. He'd had a few too many comments about his weight this past couple of days, but knew that Mr Field meant well.

'How about lunch tomorrow?' Mr Field asked. 'Don't worry—I'm not trying to fatten you up. I want to discuss something. Just us.'

'Of course,' Richard responded smoothly, even if inwardly he was a touch startled. Mr Field was busy, and in heavy demand at events such as this one.

They made arrangements—or rather Mr Field said that Tara, his secretary, would be in touch. 'Until tomorrow, then…'

Richard took the Tube to Paddington. The station was both busy and familiar. He'd been doing this journey for years, and before purchasing his ticket he stood on the concourse, looking up at the departure board and wondering if he might make the earlier train. But he saw it was just about to leave.

When somebody beside him groaned, Richard could guess why—a few trains on the board had suddenly been cancelled.

Thankfully his own was still on time.

Then the information board was updated again, and as several more trains were abruptly cancelled there was a round of collective moans.

The train to Cardiff was still on time.

Then the board was updated once more and the sign reading 'Cardiff' flipped over.

Cancelled

Richard scanned the board, looking for the later train.

Cancelled

For a second he couldn't hear the loudspeaker system, nor his disgruntled fellow travellers—or rather they all faded into insignificance as a new emotion hit him.

In his oh-so-silent way he analysed the feeling spreading in his chest as he released a long breath.

Relief.

Richard didn't ignore his feelings; he just didn't readily share them. So he had no desire to head to the rooftop bar and reveal this new development in his day, and nor did he feel the need to whip out his phone and provide a group update.

Soon he would head back to Kings Cross, but for now he simply stood there, his face impassive, silently acknowledging his internal response to his train being cancelled.

Relief.

He was relieved not to be going.

CHAPTER TWO

'Excuse me...'

Sorcha Bell's attempt to run up the escalator was once again thwarted—her petite five feet two frame and soft Scottish-accented voice had little effect on the group of people blocking her way.

'Excuse me,' she said, more loudly, and this time they parted enough that she managed to get through.

She ran the last few steps to the top, refusing to entertain the possibility that she might miss her train.

Her long red hair was whipping wildly across her face as she spilled off the escalator and raced across the concourse towards her platform. Though her lilac cheesecloth dress and cream espadrilles weren't ideal running gear, at least there was no luggage weighing her down—just a hefty overnight bag.

Making her speedy way, she was delighted to see that the platform hadn't even opened and people were still lined up.

'Made it...' she breathed, her heart hammering from her rare sprint as she joined her fellow travellers at the barrier. 'I havenae run like that since school sports day...' she said, to no one in particular.

But a breathless lady who had come up behind her laughed. 'Nor me,' she agreed. 'I was sure I was going to miss it. This is the Edinburgh train?'

'It is.' Sorcha glanced up at a Roman numeral clock that had become a frequent fixture in her life in recent months and saw that it was almost five. 'They should let us on soon,' she said, and then wondered out loud if the buffet would be open, chatting easily with the lady as the line moved.

They discussed the sultry weather, both here and at home, as well as a comedy show the lady was on her way to see.

They didn't exchange names; this was just small talk.

While Sorcha might do her best to avoid difficult conversations, when it came to small talk she excelled!

'Was he at the Fringe this year?' Sorcha checked, recognising the name of the comedian.

It was late September, and the Edinburgh Fringe Festival had been held last month. It was definitely her favourite time of the year. She lived a couple of hours out of Edinburgh, and when the festival was on she got there as often as she could.

'I'd have gone and seen him if I'd known he was playing.'

'Not this year. Apparently he—' the lady's response was abruptly terminated as a suited man collided with them, knocking Sorcha to one side.

'Hey!' the lady called out to him. 'Watch where you're going.'

Sorcha righted herself as the gentleman staggered off.

'Cheek of him,' the lady grumbled. 'Too much to drink.'

And that should have been that.

Getting her ticket ready, Sorcha moved down the line. But something was niggling, and she turned around and took another look at the man. He was middle-aged and well groomed. His neat blond hair clashed with his ruddy face and indeed he was staggering. Sorcha watched as he careered into a young man on his phone. He certainly appeared intoxicated, but as an accident and emergency nurse Sorcha knew that blaming alcohol could prove a dangerous assumption.

'Miss...?'

Someone prompted her to move along and Sorcha walked towards the barrier, about to go through. But at the last moment she looked again. The man now stood stock still as others dashed past him, and then he turned slightly and she saw him grimace and clutch his left arm.

'Miss?' a station worker called. 'Move along now, please.'

'That man...' Sorcha started, watching as the man leant forward and moved his hand from his arm to his chest.

There really wasn't time to explain. Leaving the queue, she hastily made her way towards him, hoping she was overreacting.

'Sir?'

The man was doubled over now, but he reached out and grabbed her forearm and for a second almost toppled them both. His grip was tight, and she could feel and see his desperation and panic. Sorcha knew now that she wasn't overreacting. She called out to a passerby for help, but they walked briskly on. She asked another to call an ambulance, but her voice was drowned out by the voice on the loudspeakers.

Glancing back at the clock, she saw it was two minutes after five and knew she was about to miss her train.

It didn't matter now.

'Let's get you sitting down.' She spoke as calmly as she could to the distressed man.

There were chairs a few metres away but, given that he was on the edge of collapse, they were a few metres too far from them. Instead, she managed to guide him to a wall and he leant against it, refusing to sit.

'I'll be okay,' the man insisted, trying to speak normally yet clutching his chest, his face etched with pain. 'Thank you.'

'You need to sit,' she insisted, refusing to be dismissed. 'I'm Sorcha,' she introduced herself, then told him she was a nurse and asked his name.

'Edward,' he told her. 'It's my chest…'

He started to tug at his tie, as if it was choking him, but then gave in. He seemed to accept that he could no longer stand and leant more heavily against the wall. Sorcha helped him slide down to the ground safely, turning her head and calling out as she did.

'I need an ambulance!'

Her voice was loud, the one she might use at work to summon help, but people remained oblivious, just hurrying by, or standing still and looking up at the information boards.

She was about to take out her phone and do it herself, but then the lady from the queue whom she'd chatted with was running over, and the staff member who'd been hurrying her along was coming too.

'What can I do?' the lady asked.

'Call an ambulance,' Sorcha told her, then looked to the staff member. 'Is there an AED…?'

'On to it,' he said. 'And the first aider's been called.'

'Good.'

It helped to know that someone else was on their way, and while Sorcha truly hoped she wouldn't need to use the external defibrillator, she knew Edward could go into cardiac arrest at any given second and it might very well be required.

He was seriously ill.

His face was no longer flushed. Instead it was a ghastly grey colour, and his blond hair was now dark with sweat. He was, she was sure, having a heart attack, right here and now.

'The ambulance is on its way,' Sorcha told him, and the tried to gather as many details from him as she could, such as his medical history and any allergies he suffered from. But there was nothing much she could glean. Edward's concern was for his wife.

'I'm going to have to borrow your pen,' Sorcha said, going into his jacket pocket. 'I'd never find one in my bag…'

She did have paper, though, and wrote down his contact details.

'My wife will be waiting…' He told Sorcha they were supposed to be meeting at Covent Garden. 'I'm always late.'

'It's okay,' Sorcha said, feeling his thready pulse.

'No…' He put his head back against the wall and closed his eyes. 'I'm *always* late.'

His pulse was erratic, and Sorcha could feel her own heart leaping in her chest. She was nervous and doing her best not to show it. Not for a moment did she want Edward to get a sense of her own anxiety.

Sorcha worked in an accident and emergency unit a couple of hours outside of Edinburgh, and though small it had an incredible team and all the necessary equipment. No matter the situation, she never felt alone.

Now, even though a crowd was starting to gather, she did feel alone.

Sorcha considered what best she should do if things took a turn for the worse. If Edward did arrest, she would lie him down and attach the AED when it arrived.

'Always late…' Edward muttered as she undid his tie.

'You've got a very good excuse,' Sorcha said, and then made a little joke as she removed his tie. 'I can write a sick note for you now that I've got your pen.'

He gave a small laugh as she slipped both his pen and his tie into his pocket. As was often the case, even in the worst situations a little humour helped. It didn't just help in making people smile, it drew people closer too.

Edward's eyes opened then and met her own. 'We argued about it last night,' he told Sorcha, and gave her a regretful smile.

Sorcha knew that her face might be the very last that he saw, so she forgot the crowd all gathered around and tried to ignore how scared she was.

'Do you want me to call her for you?' she asked.

'Not yet.' He shook his head. 'She suffers panic attacks.'

He was trying to protect his wife, Sorcha guessed. Trying to keep things normal for a little while longer for the woman he loved.

She heard footsteps, then a male voice. 'Here you go.' It was the staff member from before and he held an AED. Sorcha thanked him, but kept her eyes on Edward. 'The first aider's with someone else,' the man informed her as he put the AED down. 'A passenger with a severely sprained ankle. She asked how bad this is…'

'Get someone else to wait with the sprained ankle,' Sorcha said. The first aider might think this was a simple faint. 'Ask the first aider to make her way here as quickly as possible.' She turned back to Edward. 'I'm going to open your shirt,' she told him.

'You'll stay?' he checked.

'Of course.' She touched his arm. 'You're doing so well, Edward. I know you're in pain.'

How long would the ambulance take?

Glancing up at the platform clock, she was surprised to see only a few minutes had passed; it felt a whole lot longer.

And things were getting worse.

'Edward?' she said as he slumped forward.

He pulled his head up and gave her a nod, then ran his tongue over pale lips.

'Did I tell you my name?' she asked.

'Sorcha.' He nodded again. 'Scottish…?'

'Yes.'

'Our honeymoon…' He couldn't finish his sentence.

'You went to Scotland?' Sorcha said for him. 'What's your wife's name?'

He didn't answer.

'Edward?' Sorcha demanded a response. 'Tell me your wife's name.'

He stirred.

'What's your wife's name?' she asked again.

'Anna.'

She wanted to call out and ask how much longer the ambulance would be, but she didn't want Edward to hear her fear. Also, she knew it was a pointless question. It was on its way. Out of the corner of her eye she could see that the station staff were moving people back and clearing the way. They were being marvellous, really.

She still felt alone, though—especially when

Edward rallied a bit and looked at her and told her of his worry.

'I don't want to die here,' he said.

Edward's pale blue eyes met hers and she saw fear. He knew how bad this was.

'I won't let you,' she told him, and locked her green eyes with his.

It wasn't an empty promise—if he arrested, she would start CPR, and the ambulance would surely get him to hospital in time.

But then his eyes drifted away, and as suddenly things changed.

His head lolled back and his skin turned even greyer. He was diaphoretic—the sweat was pouring off him—and she undid the last buttons of his shirt, ready to attach the AED monitor, all the time speaking to him as she went.

'Sorry to be so bold…' she said, as if it was normal to be urgently stripping off a stranger's shirt. She kept talking, trying to keep the fear from her own voice. 'I'm going to lie you down now, Edward.'

'Can I help?'

She heard a deep, calm voice and looked up to see a man who immediately crouched down on Edward's other side.

'I need to lie him down.'

The new arrival nodded and took the weight of Edward's upper body. He shifted him easily and together they gently laid him on the hard floor. While this lone stranger might not be the paramedic she'd fervently hoped for, there was a quiet command to him, and Sorcha felt as if the cavalry had arrived.

'That's better,' the man said, his fingers moving to Edward's neck and taking his pulse. With his eyes still on the patient, he asked Sorcha what had occurred.

'Sudden onset of chest pain.' She glanced at the time—had it really only been that long…? 'The episode began eight minutes ago…' It truly felt like for ever.

'Has an ambulance been called?' the man asked.

'On its way.' She nodded. 'The first aider's coming, too.'

'Do you know him?'

'No. I just came upon him,' Sorcha explained. 'He was staggering…'

'Okay. Hello, sir,' he said. 'My name's Richard Lewis. I'm an emergency registrar. I work nearby.' He glanced up to Sorcha. 'Can we find an AED?'

'I've got one here.'

'Excellent,' Richard said, reaching for it and starting to attach it to Edward. He asked her name.

'Sorcha,' she told him.

The breathless first aider arrived, explaining that she'd been on the other side of the station.

'Do you have Aspirin?' Richard asked, and she nodded and went to her kit.

'Take these,' Richard said, placing them in Edward's mouth. He declined the bottle of water the first aider offered. 'They're soluble.'

'Water...' Edward gasped.

Sorcha took some gauze from the first aider's kit and doused it, then used it to moisten his lips.

There was little else they could do, yet somehow things were more calm.

Dire, yes.

But since Richard Lewis had knelt down on the other side of Edward, Sorcha had known things were completely under control. This Richard knew absolutely how to handle things, no matter the situation.

'My wife...' Edward groaned as his phone rang.

'They're supposed to be meeting,' Sorcha explained. 'He's worried about scaring her.'

'I'll speak with your wife,' Richard said as the phone rang out. But Edward shook his head, clearly still attempting to protect her.

'She suffers from panic attacks,' Sorcha said, explaining Edward's reluctance to contact his wife.

'Edward?' Richard looked him right in the eye. 'Would she want to be with you?'

He nodded.

'Then give her the chance to be.'

Edward closed his eyes and then nodded again.

'Good man,' Richard said.

'Her name's Anna,' Sorcha said as, with Edward's help, she unlocked the phone to make the difficult call.

As it rang, she handed it over to Richard.

'Anna? My name is Richard Lewis,' Richard introduced himself. 'I'm a doctor, and Edward has asked me to speak with you...' He explained the situation with a mixture of brevity and patience, his eyes never leaving Edward's face. 'It's okay. I know it's a shock,' he said into the phone. 'Take a moment—get your bearings.'

He waited a moment and then the conversation resumed, and though Sorcha knew he couldn't be certain where Edward would be taken, she heard him tell her his best guess was the hospital very close by.

'Maybe start to make your way there. We'll pass on your details to the paramedics.' He was very formal, but quietly kind. 'Yes,' Richard went on, 'he is conscious. Would you like to speak with him?'

He briefly turned away from Edward, and Sorcha heard him telling Anna to reassure Edward and to keep things calm. To let Edward know that *she* was okay.

'That will help him a lot. I'll put him on now.' He held the phone to Edward's ear. 'It's Anna...' he told him.

Edward could barely talk, but with his eyes closed he managed a few words, then added, 'I love you too.'

'She did well,' Richard told him when the call was done. 'So did you.'

All they could do now was wait and, in this awful situation, do their best to give Edward privacy and calm. There was little response from Edward now. Even so, Sorcha kept talking to him, telling him she was still here and that Anna was on her way.

'The ambulance is here,' the first aider said at last, and Sorcha sat back on her heels in relief as she looked out at the sight of the crowd parting and familiar green uniforms approaching, armed with a stretcher laden with oxygen and medical equipment.

'Richard!' one of the paramedics greeted him, clearly recognising him. 'Fancy seeing you here.'

'This is Edward...' Richard introduced the patient and Sorcha stood up to give them space to work. She was a little giddy, and her legs felt numb as she held on to the wall. The paramedics worked swiftly, taking his observations and obtaining IV access, then delivering pain control.

The ECG tracing confirmed a STEMI—a serious myocardial infarct.

'They're just letting the cardiologist at the hospital know to expect you,' Richard explained to a now very drowsy Edward as one of the paramedics transferred the tracing and liaised with a specialist.

Sorcha was used to this, albeit from the hospital end of things. The countdown started when they were alerted that an ambulance was bringing in a STEMI, and the aim was to get the patient stented within ninety minutes.

'What time did you get to him?' a paramedic asked her.

'Five,' Sorcha answered, and then recalled checking the time. 'Two minutes past five.'

Turning to look at the clock now, Sorcha was momentarily confused when she saw it was only twenty-three minutes past… She even wondered if the clock was out of order, and that the timing she'd given the paramedic might be wrong, but then Richard confirmed her timeline.

'I arrived shortly after…'

With time of the essence, and a cardiology team waiting to receive the patient, it was an utter relief when a grey-coloured and barely conscious Edward was on his urgent way to hospital. He was still breathing and his heart was still beating.

'Good job,' Richard said to the first aider, and

to all who had assisted. Then he nodded to Sorcha. 'Well done.'

'You too,' Sorcha said, smoothing down her crumpled dress and then admitting, 'I've never been so pleased to see anyone.'

'I didn't really do anything,' he said. 'You had things under control by the time I arrived.'

'Oh, no, it's always good to look up and...' She paused, unsure quite what she was trying to convey. She'd had help—the lady who had called the ambulance, and efficient staff doing all they could—but somehow, even with all those people gathered, it had been the moment Richard had arrived when she'd known things would be okay. That even if things got worse, he'd deal with it well.

Confidence?

Presence?

Sorcha decided she would think about that later; right now she had to go and see if there was any hope of making her train or transferring to the next.

'I'd better go...' She glanced up at the board. 'I've no doubt missed my train to Edinburgh, but hopefully there's another...'

'Nobody's going anywhere.' Richard halted her rapid exit. 'All the trains have been cancelled.'

'But I was just boarding...' She looked around and sure enough there was a 'Cancelled' sign above her platform and disgruntled people all around. '*All* the trains have been cancelled?'

'Apparently so.'

'When did this happen?'

'Around the time I heard you shouting for someone to call an ambulance...' He gave her a slightly curious look. 'Sorcha, are you sure you're okay?'

'I'm fine.'

'Do you want to get a drink?'

His invitation was as sudden as it was unexpected, but then she found out the reason for it.

'You're ever so pale.'

'Oh, I'm always pale...' She attempted a joke.

'No.' Richard shook his head. 'Trust me on this.'

The oddest thing was...already, she did.

Richard had seen Sorcha's slight wobble when she'd first stood, but now the colour was starting to leach from her face. Her green eyes were becoming more vivid, and the light dusting of freckles seemed to be darkening against her rapidly whitening face.

'Let's get a seat.'

He took her arm and located a café. Thankfully there was a free table outside, and he suggested she sit while he ordered for them both.

'I don't have any cash.' She took out her phone. 'But I could—'

'Sorcha,' he interrupted, 'I'd far prefer that you sit down than I have to deal with another collapse within the hour.'

'Fair enough.' Thankfully she didn't argue. 'I'll have some water...maybe a white coffee.'

He returned with far more.

'Here.' He put a tray down; there were coffees and bottles of water, as well as two baguettes. 'One's cheese and pickle; the other's chicken and lettuce. You choose.'

She first took a gulp of water, and then chose the chicken. 'Thank you so much.'

He saw she looked better just for sitting down.

'I haven't eaten all day.' She took a very grateful bite of the baguette. 'I was going to head straight for the buffet car on the train.'

'Were you in London for work?'

'No...' She shook her head. 'Just an overnight stay. I came to visit my...' She hesitated for just a second. 'My mum.'

'Doesn't she feed you?' he said, but then he saw her lips tense and realised he'd inadvertently hit a nerve. 'Sorry—that was flippant of me.'

'It's fine,' she dismissed. 'I was helping her paint, and by the time it came to lunch...' She waved a hand. 'She didnae have much in.'

'Pardon?' Her accent was strong, but aside from that he wasn't sure what she meant.

'Food-wise,' Sorcha said. 'Nothing in the cupboards or fridge. So I ended up going shopping for her. That's why I was running late.'

'I see.'

He didn't.

From what he could gather, she'd come down from Scotland to help her mother paint and had nothing to eat. Still, from her rather tense response before he knew better than to probe.

He wanted to, though, and that surprised him.

These days, outside of work, it was unusual for him to want to persist with any conversation, for no more reason than simply because...

'Do you think he'll be okay?'

Her mind was clearly still on Edward, and he dragged his attention back to the reason they were here.

'Obviously you can't say for sure, but...'

'Actually, I do think he'll be okay,' Richard said. 'At least he has the very best chance to be—the hospital is so close to Kings Cross.'

He told her a little about the hospital Edward had been taken to, and their impressive stats—how they aimed for less than ninety minutes from door to stent.

'Hopefully it will be less. I'll go and see him on Monday and find out.'

'Really?'

'Yes. I'm working in A&E there at the moment. I don't usually go onto the wards to follow up, but somehow it's more...' He considered for a moment. 'It's more personal when it happens out of work, isn't it?'

Sorcha nodded. 'It's odd...' She told him how she'd kept checking the clock. 'I honestly thought it had stopped. It felt like time slowed down.'

'When every second counts we tend to notice all of them.'

'Yes. That must have been it—every second counted.'

'You've never come across anyone ill outside of work before?' he checked.

'Never. I was terrified.'

'For what it's worth, you didn't look scared.'

'Possibly because you came along,' she admitted. 'I kept reminding myself not to show how worried I was—that I might be the last face Edward saw.'

The poignancy of her words had the small, good-natured smile Richard was wearing shifting to something more pensive. He knew Sorcha wouldn't have noticed the effect, for she was no longer looking at him, but picking at the crumbs left from her baguette.

She asked him a question.

'Where were you headed?'

'Cardiff. But all the trains from Paddington were suddenly cancelled, so I headed back to Kings Cross to find the same thing starting to happen here too. I'm here for a conference.'

'Is Cardiff not home?'

'No, I live…' He didn't get to finish, and paused as an announcement was made over the loud speakers—it didn't tell them much.

'What do you think the "foreseeable future" means?' Sorcha asked with a slight eyeroll.

'It means that I need to make a phone call,' Richard said.

'Well, I'm going to the ladies',' Sorcha said, and stood. She needed to go, but also she wanted to give him some privacy to make his call. 'Save my seat?'

'Sorry?' he checked, as if he was a little startled, or perhaps not understanding what she'd said.

'I meant I'll be back in a moment.'

'Oh…' He nodded. 'Of course.'

The loos were busy, and as she waited in line, listening in to conversations, hearing talk of a cyber-attack and that all the national railway's computers were one by one being taken down, it became clear she might not be getting home tonight. There was a flutter of panic at the thought of being stuck for the night in London—really stuck. If this dragged on there would be a lot of people looking for last-minute accommodation.

Checking online, she saw that the budget hotel she'd stayed in last night had two rooms left...

Better to be safe than sorry.

The queue took for ever.

Her good-looking coffee companion would be wondering where she'd got to, Sorcha thought as she washed her hands.

And he *was* good-looking.

Her hands paused beneath the stream of water. Now the adrenaline had faded, and now she'd had something to eat—and possibly because now she was well away from him—it dawned on her how very handsome Richard Lewis actually was.

Imagine asking someone as stunning as him to save her seat. He'd probably taken out his phone in the hope that she'd get the hint and leave, now that she was recovered.

She looked in the mirror and saw the blush she usually had while talking to someone as utterly gorgeous as him materialise.

The horror!

Her hair was wild, somehow the dust on the platform had transferred to her cheeks, and her dress was pulled down, exposing the flesh-coloured strap of her bra.

Yikes!

She splashed her face with water and then took

out a hair tie and piled her hair on the top of her head. She rearranged her dress and, looking and feeling a little more together, stepped out onto the concourse. She made her way back to the café, determined to be a little more sophisticated this time around.

If he was still there.

She was quite certain he'd be gone.

Sorcha didn't attribute the sudden feeling of dread that descended upon her to his not being there—after all, they'd barely spoken. It was a feeling she was familiar with—as if she'd been given up on...that she wasn't good enough for people to want her around.

It was a general fear of being abandoned.

It was the reason she tended to jump ship first in relationships, preferring to end things before they could be ended.

It was the very reason she was in London, trying to work things through with her birth mother in an attempt to fix herself.

Her eyes scanned the café, saw the empty table, the waiter clearing cups and plates. But just as she accepted that he was gone—the very second she thought she'd been proved right—the waiter moved and she saw Richard stepping out from inside the café. Nodding to the waiter, he retook his seat at the cleared table.

He was still there.

CHAPTER THREE

'Hey...'

Richard smiled as she approached the table and her stomach went tight. How on earth had she sat so casually with him?

'I thought you'd be gone,' Sorcha admitted as she sat.

'Why? You asked me to save your seat.' He pushed a bag towards her and she saw that in it were two almond croissants. 'I got these,' he said, loosening his tie and undoing the top button of his shirt. 'I just spoke with the waiter—it would seem we might be here for a while. Apparently it's a cyber-attack, it's happening nationwide—Birmingham now.'

'I saw on my phone.'

Richard appeared to be relaxing, yet she felt awkward for the first time—not that he seemed to notice, pulling apart a croissant as he said, 'At least you can stay with your mother.'

'I don't really know her well enough,' Sorcha sighed. But then she saw his slight frown as he glanced over and realised how odd that must sound. 'She's my birth mother. We've only very recently reconnected.'

'Oh.'

'It's probably best that I don't land on her. I don't think she'd...' Sorcha halted. This gorgeous stranger didn't need to know the details—he was simply being polite. 'Anyway, I've just booked a hotel.'

'Already?'

'I got stuck overnight in Edinburgh once without accommodation,' she told him. 'It was awful.'

Sorcha knew she was frowning now, watching as he dunked his croissant into his coffee. 'Yuck!'

'I apologise. I usually save that revolting habit for home.' He put down the soggy croissant. 'It's my one vice.'

'Well, don't stop on my account.' She got back to her reason for booking a hotel so fast. 'I didn't want a repeat of that cold night in Edinburgh, so I quickly booked a room at the place I stayed last night.'

'Fair enough—though it's a pity. I've got a hotel room nearby you could have had.'

'Dr Lewis!' She forgot to be awkward and spoke as she would to a friend, interrupting in feigned shock. 'We've only just met!'

'No, no...' He hastily moved to correct the misunderstanding, but in that same second obviously saw the gleam of humour in her eyes. He suddenly laughed. 'What I *meant*,' he said, and their eyes held as he continued, with a smile now in his tone, 'is that I'm in the middle of a conference, so I've not only got my home to go to, but a hotel room.'

'Phew!' she said as if she'd really thought for a second that this very formal man was propositioning her.

'You don't seem too bothered by the delay,' he commented after a while.

'I'm not,' Sorcha admitted. 'At least not now I've got a place to stay. I might even do a tour. I've never seen Big Ben or Buckingham Palace. I'm only ever here on short trips and always rushing back and forth…'

'And me,' he admitted. 'At least lately.'

'Was it important?'

He frowned at her question, not understanding what she was asking.

'Your trip to Cardiff?' she said.

'Yes,' he said, then swallowed. It was his absolute priority, and had been for the past three years now. But then he thought of the relief he'd felt when he'd seen the signs at Paddington flick over to 'Cancelled'.

Sorcha didn't need to hear about that. As well, he was tired of people trying to say the right thing, and weary of awkward, strained conversations—and that was exactly what this would become if he told her the truth…

Richard liked how they were now.

'I'll get there soon enough,' he said.

It was quite freeing to sit at a busy station and watch the world go by…have a slow, unfolding conversation in such pleasant company.

'Is it a big conference?' she asked.

'Huge. It's taking place over four days.'

'Do you get lots of CPD hours for it?' she asked, her eyes lighting up at the prospect of amassing continuing professional development hours.

Somehow that made him smile.

'Absolutely!' He nodded. 'That was the main reason I agreed to attend, but it's actually fired me up.'

'Worth it, then?'

'Yes.'

They chatted a bit about work, but for Richard the nicest thing was simply sitting there, at times in companionable silence and at other times sharing observations.

They even invented a new game: Phone or Passer-By.

The rules were simple and the unwitting contestants were quietly observed.

'Here comes another one…' she said now, and they both sat up and watched a woman in a smart trouser suit running from the Underground, dashing for the train she clearly thought she was about to miss, just as Sorcha had done.

'Phone!' Sorcha got her verdict in first, even before the lady had skidded to an abrupt halt.

They'd played this game several times now, and whoever declared first gave the other contestant the second choice.

They watched as the lady looked up at the information board, then slowly looked around.

'Damn,' Richard said as the lady went into her bag.

'Told you...' Sorcha said, confident that the woman's first response would be to check her phone.

'Hold on...' Richard warned.

It wasn't quite a World Cup penalty shoot-out, but there was definitely a shared vested interest as they watched the lady, phone in hand, walk towards a group of people.

'Come on...' Richard urged. 'Ask.'

'No, check your phone,' Sorcha said, 'Call someone.'

'Whoa...' Richard said, as at the last minute the lady did an abrupt turn.

They were both wrong. The lady went straight to the line up at the information booth and neither asked a passer-by nor used her phone.

A first.

It was the very nicest of delays.

'I remember that...' Sorcha nodded as a large group went by, the women in pretty dresses, the men in suits, all laughing and chatting.

'What?'

'That Friday night feeling.'

'What feeling?'

'Freedom.' She smiled. 'When the working week is done and there's nowhere you need to be. I used to work in an office.'

'Before you went into nursing?'

'It was awful,' she admitted. 'We ran out of that office on a Friday like it was the end of term break-up for the summer holidays.'

He smiled at her description.

'We miss out on that,' she said. 'Us shift workers. There was something nice about all finishing at the same time as everyone else at work.'

'True...' He thought back for a moment. 'When I was at med school, yes...the weekend was the endgame.'

Their conversation paused often, but they would sit in companiable silence for a while and then easily resume, often picking up where they'd left off.

'There are benefits to shift work,' Sorcha said now. 'Like being able to book dental appointments on a weekday and never being stuck in the rush hour.'

'I'm always getting stuck in the rush hour,' Richard sighed. 'On the Underground.'

'I might find out for myself soon,' Sorcha said. 'I had a couple of interviews last week. I'm hoping to come and work in London—just for a few months. I want to get some more experience living in the big city and all that.'

Another stretch of silence.

Then, 'What about Edinburgh or Glasgow?' Richard asked. 'They're both big and much closer to home.'

'Maybe, but...' She sighed.

Silence.

'I'd like to get to know her a bit better.'

'Your birth mother?' Richard checked, and found he had stopped looking out to the crowd and had turned to face her.

'Amanda,' she told him, and then swallowed, as if she'd surprised herself by how easily she'd told him. 'I actually call her by her name. I just said "my mum" to you because...' She offered a small shrug. 'Well, it was just easier. I didnae know we'd be talking for so long. Well, not properly talking...' She paused. 'I can't really mention her at home.' She shrugged. 'It upsets them.'

'Your adoptive parents?' he checked, and she nodded.

'Do they know you're here today?'

'No.' She shook her head. 'I just find it easier not to say.'

And for Richard it was usually that way too. It was much easier to leave things alone and not delve. Unless he was working, or coming across cardiac patients collapsed at a train station, he generally didn't get involved, and he chose never to prolong conversations. Yet there was something about being suddenly stranded with her, their paths crossing…

Something about Sorcha that made him not merely offer an ear but want to know.

And now Richard was the one who invited further conversation. 'Easier for whom?'

'All of us—my parents don't want to hear about it and I don't want to say.' She gave a small laugh. 'I'm well and truly caught now, though.'

'How so?'

'I'm supposed to be picking up my sister from the airport tomorrow. When I tell my parents I'm stuck in London it won't take them long to work out where I've been.'

'Do you live with them?'

'Gosh, no. I have my own place. They're just…'

He watched the column of her throat as she swallowed, and then she gave an uncomfortable shrug.

'I'll come up with something.'

'Perhaps you could say that you were meeting

some guy for dinner before the trains all went down?'

She gave a good-natured laugh at his unhelpful suggestion, but as she looked away he found his breathing had stilled, and he realised he might not just be offering an excuse for her parents.

Was he offering her dinner? With him?

'I'm not sure they'd buy it.' Sorcha turned to him and smiled. 'It's a long way to come for dinner.'

Richard flicked that excuse away. 'Tell them he's good company.'

'Indeed, he is,' she agreed.

'We can go for a drink first.'

'Sounds perfect.'

It was, after all, Friday night.

And there was that feeling…

Freedom. With nowhere you needed to be.

And time was doing that odd thing again.

Every second counted.

CHAPTER FOUR

IT WAS A slice of London Sorcha had never seen before.

Thankfully, Richard knew where they were headed, and soon they were walking down a little lane. Turning off it, they came to a small, very ancient-looking pub.

'I'd never have known it was here,' she said.

It was packed, as well as tiny.

'There's a garden,' he said, pointing to a doorway.

'I'm getting these drinks,' Sorcha said. 'You find us a table. What will you have?'

She carried their drinks outside, to where he'd found a gorgeous table near a tree, and put them down. 'You're a cheap date,' she said, and smiled.

There was icy white wine for Sorcha, and sparkling water with ice and lemon for Richard.

It wasn't a date. Sorcha had to keep reminding herself of that. They were here by mutual inconvenience. Biding their time until the trains got back on track, so to speak…

Yet there was a flutter in her stomach…a giddy, delicious feeling as they faced each other. They were both leaning forward now, Sorcha's elbows on the table, her chin resting on her hand as they chatted.

'So, you worked in an office,' Richard said. 'Doing what?'

'Mainly on Reception.' She groaned at the memory. 'Then they hauled me off of that because I spoke too much to the clients. It wasnae as if I was offering financial advice. It was an accounting firm in Edinburgh, and it was all very conservative and formal. We didn't have a uniform, as such, but we had to wear all greys and navy and…'

'You like fashion?'

'No, it's not that…' She couldn't really explain it. 'It was just very dour; the men all dressed in suits and ties and…' She glanced across the table at him, dressed impeccably in a suit and tie. 'I wasn't implying…' She swallowed.

'Go on.'

'Well, you look very nice in a suit.'

'Thank you.'

'And I'm sure you're not…'

'Not what?'

He'd clearly noticed her blush, and he was smiling at her discomfort, toying with her.

'Conservative.'

'Oh, but I am,' he said happily, owning it.

'All I'm trying to say is that office life wasn't for me, but I had no idea what I wanted to do back then.'

'None at all?'

'Nope.' She thought back. 'A secret agent, perhaps, a spy...' She started to laugh. 'Honestly, I had no clue. My sister always knew she wanted to be a flight attendant...' She rolled her eyes.

'What's your sister's name?' he asked.

'Theresa—she's a year younger than me.'

'And how old are you?'

'Guess.'

Richard shook his head. 'I'm not that foolish.'

'Go on,' she insisted. 'Guess.'

How old *was* Sorcha? Richard wondered. And he found it was nice to wonder about her.

She'd told him that she'd worked in an office before training as a nurse. Everything pointed towards her being mid to late twenties, but now he looked for visual clues.

Really looked.

She wore no make-up. Her lips were full, and currently parted to reveal a white, slightly toothy smile that was endearing. The blaze of wild red curls which had first caught his eye had been tied up, but stray wisps danced around her full cheeks and the low evening sun brought out the copper and gold tones.

He took in her unpierced ears, then a sweep of

his eyes over her face and neck confirmed that she wore no jewellery. His eyes drifted down, taking in her slender frame and the pretty lilac dress. He'd politely ignored the flash of lacy bra when she'd been dealing with Edward, and he very deliberately didn't allow his gaze to go there now—just came back to the green eyes that awaited his verdict.

Beautiful.

Rather than saying that, Richard chose a far more sensible response. 'Twenty-four.'

'I'm guessing you took a couple of years off to be safe?'

He smiled at her perceptiveness. 'Twenty-six, then?'

Those curls resumed their wayward dance as she shook her head. 'I'm twenty-eight.' She took a sip of her wine. 'What about you?'

'Guess,' Richard responded, when usually he wouldn't play such silly games.

It was Sorcha's turn now...

Sorcha, already a little flushed from his slow perusal, now had absolute permission to stare.

His face was elegant, with a very straight roman nose and just a slight shadow on his jaw. His hair was a dark caramel colour, with no visible flecks of grey. She took in the little fan of lines around dark blue eyes, though just for that moment she chose not to linger there. His mouth was perfection, and she tried not to wonder how it might feel to be kissed by him.

She'd never be so lucky as to know, Sorcha was sure.

Even his swallow was sexy, she decided as she watched the bob of his Adam's apple in his long neck. And finally she met the eyes that seemed so kind, and also rather wise, as if those blue depths had seen a lot.

What was the question? Oh, yes...

She hazarded a guess. 'Thirty-five?'

His gorgeous blue eyes widened in surprise. 'Correct.'

'Oh!' She let out a little laugh, and their eyes remained locked, and it was so warm and delicious to be held in his gaze. 'That was just luck.'

Lucky.

That was how she felt tonight.

'Do you have siblings?' she asked him.

'One sister—Gemma. She's a midwife.'

'And do you get on?'

'We do...' He thought for a moment. 'Just so long as we avoid talking about birthing babies. She's all for minimal intervention.'

'I thought about midwifery...' Sorcha nodded. 'That's what first got me into nursing. I wanted to get my general and then do midwifery. But then I did my A&E placement.'

'And you fell in love with it?'

'Not at first. I was terrified to start with—I still

am at times. But I loved the variety and the staff. I just knew I'd found what I wanted to do. What about you?' she asked. 'Did you always want to be a doctor?'

'Pretty much, although there were a couple of years when I wanted to be an astronaut.'

'Seriously?'

He nodded. 'But then I turned seven.'

'Oh!'

His humour was so dry, and delivered deadpan. It always caught her by surprise—like a delicious, unexpected treat.

Every time.

The pub garden was filling up and the mood was turning buoyant. Even when the news came through that there would be no trains running till the morning, rather than bemoaning the issue, people were laughing.

It felt a little as if the world had been put on hold.

All plans suspended.

As if the old rules no longer applied.

'I'd better call home and warn them I'm not going to get to the airport tomorrow,' Sorcha said, not bothering to walk away to make her call.

After all, Richard had come up with the lie.

Richard liked how she blushed and crossed her fingers as she lied about her London date.

'Mum, there was no need to tell you. It's just

dinner.' She gave him a smile. 'Yes, he's very nice. I'll tell you more when I see you.'

He watched her close her eyes and saw her blush deepen.

'Of course he has a name.' She paused. 'Richard.' She pulled an apologetic face. 'Look, I have to go.'

She ended the call.

'They think I have a mystery man now.' She sighed. 'But at least they don't think I'm here to visit Amanda.'

'It's a shame you can't talk about her with them.'

'I've never been able to.'

He watched as she ran a finger down through the condensation on her wine glass.

'I was always looking for her...long before I turned eighteen.'

He narrowed his eyes in curiosity.

'I used to check everyone.' She nodded to a group of new patrons arriving. 'Like those people sitting down. I used to wonder if one of the women might be her.'

'When did they tell you?' he asked, but then he added, 'Please feel free not to say. I was just...'

'Making conversation?'

'No,' he corrected. 'Enjoying our conversation.'

'And me,' she agreed. 'It's a relief to talk about it. I can't discuss it with anyone back home.'

'What about your sister?'

'No.' She shook her head.

'Wouldn't she get it more than most?'

'Theresa's not adopted. My parents couldn't have children—or they thought that was the case. Until lo and behold, just after they adopted me, Mum fell pregnant with my sister.'

'I've heard of that happening.'

'Well, it happened to them! I'm sure if they'd already had Theresa they wouldn't—'

She halted, closing her lips on what she'd been about to say, although he could guess.

'You don't think they'd have adopted you?'

'Who knows? Anyway, while Theresa's lovely now, when we were little she'd—'

Sorcha stopped talking and gave a tight shrug, about to shut the conversation down. But then she looked up to those beautiful blue eyes that were so patient and present, and she felt safe under his steady gaze.

Safe enough to speak on.

'She'd point out that I didn't look like anyone else in the family.'

He said nothing, and she was grateful for that.

'And when I was naughty…' He smiled a little at that. 'Oh, I was very naughty,' Sorcha assured him. 'Theresa would warn me that if I didn't behave, our parents would send me back.'

His smile disappeared, yet his eyes never diverted from her gaze.

'She was just a little girl. I know that. And if I brought it up now I'm sure she'd be horrified that she ever said those things, and that I remember them.'

'I can see why you might not want to talk to her about your birth mother.' He seemed to consider things for a moment, then, 'What about talking with your friends?'

'They have all known me since I was small. They know my parents too. It would feel disloyal.'

Oh, he got that. So much so that he closed his eyes for a second.

'I feel I'd be letting them down,' she said.

'Yes...' Richard reminded himself that this wasn't about him and opened his eyes. 'I can understand that.' He offered a pale smile. 'So, you give the filtered "everything's fine" version?'

'Pretty much.' Sorcha nodded.

'You're welcome to talk it through with me,' he offered. 'If that might help? Sometimes it's easier to talk to a stranger.'

'Maybe...'

Richard didn't feel like a stranger to her, though.

When he went to get another round of drinks Sorcha thought about his offer. There was something so steady about him—something she'd felt the very moment she'd looked up on the station concourse. She still didn't know if it was confidence, or presence, or quite what it was. She just knew there was *something*, even if she couldn't define it. And there was enough that she found herself wanting to open up for the first time about that which could not be spoken of at home.

Watching him walking back to their table carrying their drinks had her smile as if in a reflex action.

'It's packed in there,' he said, taking his seat opposite.

It felt peaceful out in the garden, though. Oh, there was laughter, and chatter, but little fairy lights were starting to twinkle in the trees and the dusk made it feel even more intimate.

'I don't want to bore you,' she warned. 'And I think you'll be too polite to say if I am.'

'I'm not that polite,' he said, and pointed to a beer. 'I got a pint.'

'You'll stop me…?'

'You'll know if I say I have to get my train…'

Given every train in London was out, Sorcha laughed.

'So…' He took a sip of his drink. 'How did you find out?'

'I've always known. My parents were very good about all that. I was nine months old when they adopted me. I was with Amanda for just a few weeks before she surrendered me. Then I had a short spell in a foster home. She was allowed to write and send cards and such.'

'Amanda?' he checked, and she nodded.

'She never did, though. I tried asking about her as I got older, but my mum and dad would always go quiet. When I turned eighteen, I contacted an agency. It took a while, but finally they put us in touch. We had a few phone calls, and then a meeting was arranged. Amanda lived in Manchester then. My parents wanted to come with me...'

'Did they?'

'Not quite.' She gave a wry smile. 'They just *happened* to be in Manchester that day.'

'You saw them?'

He couldn't help but smile.

'Believe me, James and Jean Bell would not make good spies.' She laughed at the memory. 'I wanted to do it by myself, but even so it was nice knowing they were close by.'

'What was meeting her like?'

'It was odd,' she admitted. 'An anticlimax. There was no rush of love or tears or anything— at least not from Amanda. I wanted answers, but I wasn't brave enough to ask the tough questions. We met a few times, and I thought we were maybe getting closer, but then she stopped taking my calls. She ghosted me, I guess.'

'That must have been hard.'

'I was a mess. But I put it all behind me...forgot about her.'

'*Did* you forget?'

His question was unexpected. Sorcha was used to the subject of her birth mother being avoided rather than probed—treated as something best not discussed—and to hear it addressed so directly had her eyes flying to his.

'No,' she admitted. 'I could never forget.' After years of denial, she found herself suddenly able to be honest. 'I made out that I'd put it behind me. But then earlier this year Amanda made contact, asking if we could meet up again. I decided it would be better not to tell my family. My boyfriend...' She saw a slight question in his eyes. 'At the time,' she added. 'Well, he advised against it.'

'You didn't take his advice?'

'No. We broke up—though not because of that.'

Richard wanted to ask why they'd broken up. He wanted to delve. Only that wasn't what they'd agreed to, and nor was it what this conversation was about.

'I've been coming to visit her once a month or so since then,' she said.

'Have you got the answers you wanted?'

'She's not very chatty.' Sorcha sighed. 'It's quite hard work.'

'Does she look like you?'

'No!' she exclaimed. 'Honestly, not a bit. I think I must take after my father—only she doesn't talk about him. My sister is a mixture of both my mum and dad... I just want to recognise myself in someone.'

'That's something I've always just taken for granted,' he admitted. 'I look like my father.'

'What about your sister? Does she look like you?'

'Yes,' he said. 'Well, she's possibly a bit prettier.'

She laughed, and it felt like a long time since he'd made someone laugh, made a small joke and just…

They were flirting.

Lightly.

He didn't know quite when that had started, but it was mutual and light and so unexpected tonight.

Any night.

Even so, he'd offered to listen, and he was good at that, so he didn't focus on her green eyes or the tiny gap between her front teeth. Instead, he focussed on what was being said.

'I don't want to hurt my parents, but I do want to get to know Amanda some more. The second I mention London, though, they get cross.'

'They're scared, maybe?'

'I don't know why; they're not going to lose me.'

'No, I mean…' He pondered for a moment. 'Are they perhaps worried that you're going to be hurt again?'

'I'm older now, though. I know it's not going to be all rainbows and unicorns.'

'I'd be worried,' Richard admitted. 'If you were mine.'

He hadn't meant to say that.

'If you were mine.'

Richard went to take a sip of beer and found his glass was empty, but he went through the motions anyway. 'If I cared about you,' he attempted, then gave a wry laugh. 'What I'm trying to say, albeit not very well, is that…'

'That I need to careful?' Sorcha finished for him. 'I intend to be.'

'Good.'

'Now I've taken up enough of your time, but thank you.' She reached for her bag, and he guessed she was a little embarrassed at revealing so much. 'You've been a very nice person to be stranded with.'

'How about that tour?' he said, and she blinked. 'We can get dinner afterwards.'

'You don't have to do that.'

'It would be my pleasure.'

They made their way to the Underground.

It was hot—baking hot—and the platform was very, very crowded.

'I need to get my bearings,' Sorcha said, and he steered her away from the masses to a large map of the Underground.

'Where's your hotel?' he asked.

'On the Piccadilly line. How do I get back there from Buckingham Palace?'

He pointed, and while she should have been listening to his instructions—heaven knew she needed them—instead she found her gaze on his hands.

He had nice hands...with long, slim fingers and neat nails. There was the glint of a watch peeking from beneath his cuff.

'Got it?' he checked.

'No,' she admitted with a laugh.

'It's quite straightforward.'

'For you, maybe.'

She looked at the knot of coloured lines and wished she was like the woman who came up next to her now and gave the map a cursory glance. Then, clearly satisfied that she now knew where she was going, she turned and walked off. No matter how patiently Richard explained, Sorcha couldn't get it.

'I was the same as a student,' she admitted. 'We'd all stand around an X-ray, everyone nodding...'

He laughed. 'I'm sure you weren't the only one just nodding along.'

'That's true,' she agreed. 'Where do you live?'

'Canary Wharf.' He pointed to the map.

'Why are you staying at a hotel near Kings Cross, then?'

'To be sociable at the conference,' he said. 'But I changed my mind.'

* * *

Richard turned to face her, casually unprepared for the fact that the world as he knew it was about to fall away.

For the first time in the longest time he was exactly where he wanted to be.

Sorcha smiled her slightly toothy smile and he felt the thump of his heart. It felt as if, after the deepest sleep, his body had returned to life.

He breathed in air that tasted as clear and delicious as if he'd been hauled half drowned from a lake.

He'd known she was gorgeous, and had accepted the physical attraction. Right from the start that had been undeniable—albeit a jolt to his senses. He'd felt dead inside for a very long time, after all. The real surprise was their connection. It was something way more than physical.

He wanted to explain to her just how incredible these few hours had been.

How he felt like himself again.

No matter how others tried, he always felt sequestered from them. But now he looked into green eyes that weren't clouded with sympathy or averted with awkwardness. Instead it felt as if they were looking right into him.

A different him, though. A new him. One who Richard himself didn't yet know.

He didn't do silly things like sit at a train station and people-watch with a woman he'd just met.

Never had.

Until tonight.

And he wasn't one for going to see Buckingham Palace on a whim.

Nor to sit with someone, digging up long-ago dreams of being an astronaut.

And nor did he kiss women on crowded tube platforms. But he was thinking about doing exactly that now.

'I'm very glad I changed my mind,' he admitted now.

For had he gone back to the hotel he'd be eating there now, or out eating a curry, and he didn't even know if that remained his favourite.

'I'm glad you did too,' Sorcha said.

The whoosh of an approaching tube train seemed to mirror the rush in her stomach.

'We'll get the next one,' she suggested when a packed tube came in.

But Richard just laughed.

'I don't think they'll get any better while all the mainline trains are down.'

Together they squeezed on.

It really was packed, but Richard held a handle, and Sorcha held his arm, and she'd never felt more comfortable with anyone. Only that wasn't quite right. Because when the tube lurched, and so too did Richard, she felt his free hand briefly on her arm, just steadying her, and the warmth of his touch remained long after the source had been removed.

His scent was light, and clean, and he was nothing like anyone she'd been attracted to before or dated.

Not that any of those relationships had worked out.

Sorcha had never allowed anyone close enough.

She really was brilliant at small talk, though. So good that no one could ever guess they were being shut out.

She didn't feel that way tonight.

'Here we are...' Richard said as the train swished to a stop.

As they surfaced above ground her arm was still tingling from that brief touch. And as they walked she had to keep reminding herself that this wasn't a date...that her tour guide was temporary and merely being polite.

'Look at it!'

She smiled at the sight of the palace ahead of them, softly lit, but nonetheless a strong, solid presence quietly beckoning them closer.

'It's stunning,' Richard agreed. 'I haven't been up this way in years. I think when you live near something you tend to take it for granted.'

'I don't.' She looked over at him and quashed that theory. 'When I'm in Edinburgh, no matter what I'm doing, I look up and see the castle... Or when I'm getting the train I look at it again, as we come in to Waverly...still there, always there. And I just... Well, my heart squeezes. Every time.'

'Really?'

He paused, slowed right down, and for a little while they stopped walking and faced each other.

'Absolutely,' she said. 'Don't you come here for picnics? Or when there's something big on?'

'Picnics?' He shook his head. 'No, I'm always working, or...'

'That's an excuse,' she protested.

He smiled.

'Often I take myself to the botanical gardens and I just—' She stopped. Not because he'd interrupted her, but because there was nothing to say right now. She just wanted to acknowledge the pleasure of being with him on this unexpectedly gorgeous night. 'Thank you for bringing me here.'

Their eyes met, and while she still couldn't work out their exact shade of blue, she felt it was one she already knew.

'It's my pleasure,' he said.

They walked the short distance remaining towards the palace, and then she tripped—possibly because she had three-inch wedges on, or more likely because she was daydreaming and not properly paying attention to her surroundings.

'These shoes…' she moaned.

'Here,' Richard said and offered her his arm.

It was a first for Sorcha.

This whole night was something else completely.

Quite what it was, she didn't know.

He was quiet, as if deep in thought. Was he wrestling with something? Or maybe he was bored with his companion now?

Richard was far from bored.

He was miles from where he'd intended to be, and yet he felt as if he was in precisely the right place.

He looked down and gave her a smile.

Buckingham Palace was everything Sorcha had hoped it would be—beautifully illuminated and bathed in a soft glow. Though unfortunately she had to let go of Richard's arm to get adequately close and peer through the bars. She looked up at the oh-so-familiar building, larger in real life than she'd imagined.

'What time do they change the guards?' she asked.

'I have no clue,' Richard admitted. 'I'm not sure if they do it at night.'

'You're not a very good tour guide,' she teased, and glanced over at him. 'Actually, you're a lovely tour guide—just not very knowledgeable about times and things.'

'Had I known my tour guide services would be required tonight I'd have planned accordingly.'

'Really?' She turned to face him.

'Really,' he confirmed. 'I'll do better next time.'

Their eyes met and she stared up at this very assured man who now seemed a touch bemused—as if he couldn't quite believe they were talking about there being a 'next time'.

'Listen...' he said.

She frowned, but then heard the low chimes that were so familiar from the television.

'Big Ben...' she breathed, and in the still, windless night there were ten chimes.

She heard and felt each one, while gazing into eyes whose colour she still hadn't worked out. And again she felt she knew.

There was another low chime and she realised it was eleven, and that she'd utterly lost track of time. 'I should be pulling into Waverly now...' she said, and he nodded.

'With your heart squeezing?' he said, repeating what she'd said while gazing at her as if he knew that her heart actually was squeezing right now.

She'd thought she must be imagining the attraction, or dreaming and wishing, but every molecule in her body flared as his hand lifted and he brushed her hair back from her face.

To kiss and be kissed felt as necessary to her as breathing. There was no question, no hesitation. It was as if the ache to know each other's lips simply had to be answered.

His kiss was light, and it felt like a stroking deep inside. It felt like a precursor…a little warning that if a light kiss could evoke such a warm stirring, then what else could it do?

She parted her lips to find out, and felt his shiver as he slipped his tongue inside her mouth.

They sank into each other, aching for each other. Her hands moved to the back of his head, not just to feel his hair, or press his face to hers, but so their bodies could be closer.

Their tongues mingled as they breathed in each other and tasted each other and got lost in each other.

She had never thought a kiss could be so delicious. Nor considered that one day she might stand outside a palace and feel she might as well be in a field, because it was as if the only people here were them.

They both pulled their heads back for a second, their eyes meeting almost in a frown of surprise. Because this really was heaven.

Then they were straight back to deeper kisses, to a slight moan from him, and heat from the press of his hands. And the warmth of the evening was nothing compared to the heat between them.

Then Richard pulled back again, and she knew it was only to stop himself from pulling her indecently closer into him.

She leant her head on his chest and looked up to the palace balcony, where so many kisses had been had. He made her feel like a princess. And this magical kiss told her that something incredible really was taking place.

'What do you like to eat?' he asked suddenly. 'We're probably a little late for a restaurant...'

He halted, because of course food had long since lost its importance.

Sorcha was still leaning on him a little, and she felt him pull her in closer, breathe in the citrussy coconut fragrance of her hair.

'I don't know if I want anything to eat,' she admitted.

It was odd not to be able to locate all her senses. Not to know if she was hungry, or if the ache clutching at her stomach and the craving within her was simply desire.

'Can we go back to your hotel?' she asked.

'Are you sure that is what you want?' he checked, and his hand cupped her cheek.

She nodded. 'Completely.'

CHAPTER FIVE

SORCHA HAD NEVER done anything like this in her life—only it didn't feel reckless. They kissed some more on the Underground platform and then sat on the tube train, staring at their reflection in the window opposite their seats.

Hand in hand they walked to his hotel, with pauses for more kisses along the way and one little stop at a store, because Richard had the forethought to make sure they had protection.

Sorcha stood outside as Mr Sensible went in to make his purchase. Usually, she was sensible when it came to sex, she thought, as a fire engine raced by. Its sirens and lights seemed to match how she felt on the inside. Not even sensible, she reflected. In truth, she'd always found sex a bit underwhelming.

Not tonight.

'Come on, you,' Richard said, and now there was no more stopping for kisses—not with a lovely bed so close by. They speed-walked the last few metres, and then crossed the hotel foyer and reached the elevators.

'Hurry up,' she said, as the elevators slowly descended. 'Or we could always take the stairs.'

'It's here,' he said, and she almost folded in relief at the prospect of being alone with him.

But not quite yet.

The opening doors revealed a dark-haired woman who gave him a delighted smile. 'Richard!' she exclaimed as she stepped out.

'Hi, Monica.'

'I thought you were heading to…?'

Her voice trailed off when she saw Sorcha, and Sorcha felt the cast of the other woman's eyes and saw both the surprise and curiosity in them.

Even standing apart, she and Richard must be so lit with passion that Monica immediately got that they were together.

'Oh, yes, the trains… I heard about that.' Monica wished them goodnight and walked off.

'That was awkward,' Sorcha said when the lift doors had closed. 'I don't think your friend approved.'

'It's fine. She's just…'

Richard had seen the flare of surprise in Monica's eyes, and really, he couldn't blame her for it.

It was most out of character—at least it was for the Richard that Monica knew.

'Just what?' Sorcha asked.

But he pulled her back into his arms and the little niggle was doused by contact.

'Surprised,' he said. 'But there's no need for her to be. We both know what's happened between us tonight,' Richard said, and then kissed her again.

The oddest thing was that his words, to Sorcha, made utter and complete sense.

They both knew that something special had happened tonight.

And they both wanted what was about to happen...

The suite was large and softly lit, the bed vast, with the covers turned back.

'The fairies have been in,' Sorcha breathed.

And the fairy dust must still be in the air, for modesty was gone, and both of them were stripping off with as much haste and lack of inhibition as they might if a gorgeous lake beckoned.

Only it wasn't a lake. It was a huge white bed and they dived into it together, then lay naked, facing each other, their limbs knotted, still in discovery... Touching, kissing, exploring...

Richard was as exquisite undressed as dressed—or rather, more so. His body was toned, and Sorcha traced a finger over his dark red nipples.

'I'm so pale,' she said, because her areolae were barely visible.

But he kissed them, and sucked them, and it didn't matter if the pink barely showed. His mouth on her breasts was both soft and yet thorough, his tongue, the sucking, the pressure tightening her inside.

'You're perfect,' he said.

She ran a hand down one long arm, then moved it back to his cheek. 'So are you.'

'I want you so much… But I want…'

She was holding his fierce erection and stroking it, wanting to touch him and know him, but at the same time wanting him inside her.

'I know…'

She wanted to linger on the feel of his fingers as he stroked her thigh, and on how they were both beyond waiting for this union, and yet she was desperate to explore, for them to know each other, as if every touch mattered.

Deeply, it did.

Sorcha hated the red curls between her legs. He adored them.

He explored her, stroking her with his fingers, and her lips were reaching for his mouth, suddenly desperate as he stroked her within.

But then he removed his hand. 'I want to taste you.'

'I don't…'

She attempted to protest as he moved and knelt

between her thighs. She hadn't thought she could ever enjoy anyone going down on her.

'I'm going to come the minute I'm inside you... you turn me on so,' he said.

And she looked at him, indecently erect, and reached for him.

'And I'm going to come the second you're in,' Sorcha said. Her legs were shaking, and she was taut with desire as she held the velvet skin and stroked him, then ran a finger over his moist tip. 'So you don't have to.'

'*Have* to?' he checked. 'Sorcha, believe me, I want to.'

He moved her hand away, met her eyes as he rolled on a condom. And then, unperturbed, he moved down the bed and lay on his stomach.

'I might have to fake it,' she warned.

He laughed. She felt his breath on her hot, swollen sex, and then that perfect mouth grazed softly upon her.

She moaned as he explored her...fingers, mouth and tongue all concentrated so thoroughly on her. The low noises he made had her weakening. And then his hands took her hips and he pressed her in.

'Oh, God...' Even the soles of her feet were curling on his back as she came to his lips.

A considerate lover would give her time to recover, she thought as he moved over her. But she preferred him inconsiderate and taking her swiftly, while she was still hot and swollen.

The weight of him was delicious...warm...and he was moving above her and firing her from within. He filled her, stretched her and moved with her, slowly at first. She angled her hips, met his thrusts. She knew he was holding back, as if he was fighting not to come, but she simply didn't care.

Both satisfied and suddenly desperate, she was taut, and tension was building within her again. Richard moved to his elbows, his pace more rapid, and now he was no longer holding back.

She moaned, and it was a sound she'd never made before. 'Oh...' She was urgent, wanting more of this sensation, her every nerve warm and tingling, alive in a way they had never been.

Now their ardour was deeper, and she knew they both relished the mesh of their hot bodies.

It did not feel transient...more like a deepening. They were brand-new to each other, but so in tune, locked into each other. It was as if time had lost all meaning when the cyber-attack had come, and while they might have known each other only for a matter of hours, had shared only a little history, their bodies were old lovers and friends.

Richard sank into sensation, and then looked into her eyes, felt her hand on his cheek. He moved deep within, watching her closely... He saw the way she bit her lower lip and then, when he moved again, saw her neck start to arch. He felt the lift of her hips and the warmth of her tightness around him.

He'd never known such pleasure, nor that he could feel so desperate as he drove her closer to the edge. He upped the tempo, and as her body stretched, arched upwards, she constricted below him and he felt the beckoning of her orgasm, her slight cry as he swelled and released into her.

They lay in the dark place they'd made together, him still on top, her dragging in air and holding his shoulders. He felt disorientated, but nicely so, as if they'd been somewhere and had now returned.

'Damn,' Richard said.

And even as Sorcha fathomed the change to his tone she felt the warm, wet trail as he pulled out and knew why—the condom had torn.

But what could have been a wretched moment was otherwise—as if nothing could invade the bliss they'd just experienced. They even kissed for a moment, still a little dizzy from pleasure, with their bodies still warm and close. So much so that she grumbled when he rolled off.

Sorcha lay still, thirsty for water, but too sated to move.

'Are you okay?' he asked, when the useless condom had been taken care of.

'Thirsty,' she admitted. 'But apart from that…'

He handed her a bottle of water and undid the lid of his own, and now she felt utterly content as they put down their drinks and then lay facing each other.

He addressed what had happened. 'Sorry about that.'

'Please don't worry. I am on the pill.'

'We should have been more careful.'

'We were careful.' She smiled. 'Maybe you should go back to the shop and ask for a refund.'

His hand was stroking her arm, their heads were on the same pillow, and there was so much happiness in the air she felt as if she could reach out and grab a handful.

She had never stared into the eyes of another person so readily.

So blatantly.

Now she knew their colour.

They were lighter than navy.

Twilight blue, if there was such a shade.

They reminded her of the night sky in Scotland at summer solstice…on one of those nights when the sun never really set and light was always on the horizon.

It wasn't a night for sleeping, even though they

were so late to bed, so they lay talking and wating for the dawn.

'I wonder how Edward's doing?' said Sorcha.

'I'll call and find out soon,' Richard said. 'I might have to take him some flowers on Monday to thank him.'

Sorcha laughed. 'I should check and see if the trains are running.'

'Hopefully not.'

'You've got your conference,' she reminded him.

'I do. And I'm meeting someone for lunch. A consultant I trained under.'

'Well, you can't miss that.'

'I know. Do you have to go back this morning?'

'I don't know.'

It seemed an odd answer, but her real life felt so far removed from now that she had to cast her mind out to actually recall a world that wasn't just them.

'I'm supposed to be going out with Beth tonight.' They were so close she felt as if he should know these details already. 'She's a good friend.'

'Would she understand if you couldn't make it?'

'She would,' Sorcha agreed.

But the thing was, she didn't quite understand herself. She was lying in bed with a man she'd met only yesterday, cancelling plans, putting everything on hold for more of this.

If felt perfect, though, apart from her stomach growling.

'I need food. That baguette seems a very long time ago.'

'It's all you ate yesterday.'

'I think Amanda forgot I was coming.' She knew he saw the slight pinch of her lips but he didn't say anything. His hand remained on her arm, though. 'Usually I visit once a month—it's cheaper to book in advance—but she asked me to help with some painting.' She frowned. 'Or maybe I jumped in and offered. I just want…'

Sorcha paused, unsure how to explain how she wanted the fear inside herself to abate. How she hoped if she sorted things with her birth mother it might help fix herself. Because she'd never felt good enough—always sure that if anyone got close they'd soon tire of her and leave. Not just men, but friends when she was growing up and her parents and sister.

Yet here she lay, in bed with a man she'd just met, and she was on the edge of baring the darkest parts of her soul.

No.

'I just want to establish some sort of a relationship with her, I guess,' she said instead.

'Fair enough.' Richard nodded.

'What time do you have to go down?' she asked.
'Nine...'

But when she wrapped seductive arms around his neck and pressed her body to his, he unwrapped them.

'Why don't we get room service for breakfast?' he suggested.

There was something Richard needed to share with her. And he knew the conversation to be had should take place out of bed.

He picked up the menu and they ordered a relative feast.

'Freshly squeezed juice? Coffee or tea?' he asked, then smiled. 'White coffee?'

They were starting to know the little things about each other.

When she couldn't decide between granola with the yoghurt or compote, he ticked both. Then there was a full English breakfast for him, pancakes for Sorcha.

He used the bedside phone to call in the order.

'I'm going to have a quick shower,' he told her.

'Can you call the hospital first?' she asked. 'Find out about Edward? I doubt they'd tell me anything.'

It wasn't that straightforward.

The night staff hadn't been involved with Edward's care, but after a few moments he was put through to CCU and connected to someone he knew.

'Judy, it's Richard Lewis...' He explained what had happened the day before, and paused for a moment as Judy spoke, offering to go and find out. 'I'd appreciate that.'

He squeezed Sorcha's thigh through the sheet as he waited, and finally Judy returned.

'That's marvellous news,' he said.

The news was indeed wonderful.

'Edward's currently sitting up in bed having a cup of tea,' he told Sorcha. 'And apparently Anna was there at the hospital when he arrived.'

It sounded as if Judy had spoken with Edward himself before passing the news on, and clearly he was doing incredibly well.

'I'm going to have that shower now,' he said. 'Save my seat.'

Sorcha laughed, knowing he was referring to yesterday, and lay in bed, hearing the shower being turned on. She had not even a tinge of regret. She was just bathed in pure bliss. Sure, there would be plenty of questions from her parents about this mystery man, and she'd have to cancel Beth and she felt bad about that, but for now they felt like little pebbles on a gorgeous expanse of beach.

It was easily the most relaxed she had felt in a very long time—if ever. Excited too, for the day ahead, but so relaxed that when the bedside phone rang, rather than ignore it, or call out to him, she simply answered it, assuming it was the kitchen with a question over their breakfast order...they had ordered rather a lot.

'May I speak with Dr Lewis?'

'Erm...' Sorcha glanced at the bathroom door and could hear the water still running. 'He's not available right now.' It was only then that she wished she hadn't picked up the phone. 'Can I take a message?'

'I really do need to speak directly with him. It's regarding his wife...'

Sorcha almost dropped the receiver. She felt as if she'd been thumped, or as if she'd plummeted from a great height. 'His wife?'

Richard had a wife!

She caught sight of herself in the long mirror opposite the bed, saw her own horrified expression and, worse, saw the bed she sat in, all rumpled from their lovemaking.

She didn't know how to respond to the caller—what on earth could she possibly say?—and so instead of responding she abruptly hung up the phone.

As if she were guilty.

As if she'd been caught.

'No.' She shook her head, as if to clear it, and tried to convince herself that there had been a mix-up, that whoever had called had got things wrong...

Yes. She leapt at that thought, clung onto it. There had to be a mistake, a mix-up—or was she being naïve?

Her eyes lit on his wallet, lying closed on the bedside table. She glanced at the bathroom door and then picked it up.

Trembling, she peeled apart the leather, her heart sinking when she saw a photo. Stifling a sob, she stared into his smiling, lying eyes and then turned her attention to his very beautiful bride, with her clouds of dark hair and velvety brown eyes and a smile on her face as bright as the summer sun.

'Oh, God...'

She pushed the photo down, snapped the wallet closed and stared in horror at the bathroom door. Oh, she'd love to be brave enough to confront him. To rap on the door and barge in, ask what the hell? But the man she'd thought she had met wasn't behind that door.

He'd lied.

Or rather, she hadn't asked the right questions.

Her tendency to avoid the tough questions was damning her now, for it made her complicit.

No, she did not want a showdown. All she felt was guilt and shame, and an utter fool for succumbing to his charms.

It took her seconds to dress.

A minute at the most.

She pulled on her knickers, half did up her bra and tugged on her lilac dress. Then with trembling hands she tied her espadrilles. Certainly, she didn't stop to sort out her hair—just collected her bag.

As she opened the door she saw there was a man there, with a huge silver trolley. Their breakfast was here.

Sorcha held the door open for him, but she couldn't even respond to his polite greeting and dashed for the elevator.

Richard knew he had to tell Sorcha about Jess.

And it didn't daunt him. Rather it amazed him. Because it was a conversation he'd never expected to have. He'd never expected to feel close enough to another woman to want to share the details of his life.

He stood under the icy water and felt invigorated—not just from the refreshing shower, but from his time with Sorcha.

Last night he'd held back from saying anything. At first because they'd just been talking, and he'd never thought they were headed for bed. And then, as the night had progressed, and as he'd wanted to keep more of her company, he'd wanted to prolong *them*.

He'd just been so sick of sympathy, of suggestions, of being told how to live his life, how he must feel...

But it had been more that.

Last night he'd felt himself.

A new self.

He'd trained himself to live in the present, to deal only with what *is*. And it had worked. Because it was hell to look back, and certainly he didn't know how to look to the future.

He wasn't even doing that now.

For the first time in what felt like for ever he was looking up. As if emerging from the darkest tunnel and taking a breath, looking around. And the world wasn't too bright after all—it was colourful, painted in gold and coppers, and it had smiling green eyes.

Wrapping a towel around his hips, he stepped out of the bathroom and saw that their breakfast was here. There was a serving trolley holding jugs of juice and silver cloches, but he barely gave it a glance as he frowned at the empty bed and took in her absence.

'Sorcha?'

Her clothes were gone. Her bag was gone.

Sorcha was gone.

Only just...

The air stirred, her fragrance lightly swirled,

and he went straight for the door, wrenching it open. But there was no sign of her in the corridor.

He wasn't about to chase anyone—and not just because he wore only a towel. Grand gestures and demands were not in his DNA. He was too level-headed for all that.

It was more than unexpected.

He felt as if the world had tipped the wrong way for a brief second and then tipped back. Only now it felt on the wrong level, or the wrong axis... just off-kilter somehow.

Even though he knew she didn't have his number he picked up his phone. Just in case she'd called.

As if in response to his bewilderment it buzzed, and for a second he thought it must be Sorcha. Thought that he was about to get an explanation—find out she'd locked herself out, or...

It was Trefor...

His father-in-law.

'Hey,' Richard said, in a voice that sounded a little off. He was staring around the room, and his feet seemed in two worlds—the one he'd just found, and the one that was the rest of his life, calling him back.

'Jess had a bad night,' Trefor informed him. 'Richard, I think you ought to get here.'

CHAPTER SIX

Fool me once...

London had possibly fooled her twice.

It had been a mistake to come.

It had been an impulse decision, and Sorcha tended only to make them when she was upset.

She'd taken the early-morning train back the morning after her night with Richard, and had leant her head against the window and gone over and over the day before. Searching for clues, for moments when she should have guessed, should have asked or should have known.

Not even the sight of Edinburgh's castle had soothed her. Instead her eyes had filled with tears when she'd thought of standing with him at Buckingham Palace.

She'd forgotten to cancel Beth, who'd wanted a big night out, and she'd sat awkwardly as Beth had been chatted up.

'What wrong wi' your friend?' Mr Awful had enquired as Sorcha had sat there a little stony-faced.

And then, a few days later, her head still spinning from her time with Richard, she'd been offered a job at The Primary Hospital in London.

Sorcha's initial response had been to reject it out of hand. But then she'd looked at things more sensibly... The offer was for a six-month contract and The Primary was in the north of London, close to where Amanda lived. It was not far from where Richard worked, but there was very little chance of seeing him—and anyway, why should she even factor Richard Lewis into her decisions?

She'd started working there at the end of October, but almost immediately after her arrival in London, Sorcha had realised the move was a huge mistake.

Things weren't going brilliantly with Amanda— she'd barely seen her since she'd arrived—and the flat-share she'd found for herself was far from ideal. Thankfully it was a month-by-month rental agreement, and she knew she should find somewhere else. But now it was the middle of November, and the days were markedly shorter. And as she trudged towards her first in a run of night shifts London felt dark, cold and lonely.

Or was it that London could never again feel as it had that night she'd spent with Richard?

Sorcha hated it that she still thought of him.

The good parts, which she'd tried to blot out,

still slipped into her dreams, or into her memory if she dared to daydream…

And now she had two weeks on nights in the busy city.

The Primary was a massive hospital, and every time she walked through the entrance it daunted her. It consisted of a central concrete tower with various modern extensions—part spaceship, Sorcha thought, and part rundown housing estate.

Unlike home, where she knew everyone, here there was an endless stream of new staff. And tonight, as she stepped into the changing room, amongst those she already knew there was another set of new faces.

'Hiya.' She smiled. 'I'm Sorcha…'

'Jane—I only work Friday nights.' The woman nodded to a colleague. 'Cindy's a regular on nights too. Who's in charge tonight?' Jane asked Cindy, checking the pockets of her scrubs for pens and such.

'May, I think. And Marcus is second in charge.'

'You know May already?' Jane checked.

Indeed, Sorcha did.

May was the Nurse Unit Manager, and had interviewed her. She was a stalwart of the department. Her Irish accent was soft, but her wit and her eyes were sharp. When she came into the changing room carrying her basket, she gave them all a smile.

'Have you seen that waiting room?' She tutted, opening up her locker. 'You'd think they all had better places to be.'

As Jane and Cindy headed out, May asked them to make her a cup of tea, then turned her attention to Sorcha, who was still changing. 'Are you looking forward to starting nights?'

'I am.' Sorcha nodded as she pulled on some scrubs.

They didn't match—the top was a dark purple, the bottoms lilac—but they were the least threadbare pair on the trolley. Even though they were sized extra small, they were still huge—so much so that Sorcha had left a T-shirt on beneath.

'We'll see if you feel the same in the morning.'

The department was busy, and there was a lot of backlog to clear as well as a constant stream of new patients coming in. Patients and their families were arriving in Reception, ambulances were pulling up, as well as more urgent cases being wheeled in.

'We are in for a night,' May warned as the team gathered at the nurses' station, and then she ran a knowing eye over the huge whiteboard that was constantly being updated. There were electronic boards also, but the staff constantly worked from the central one, updating it themselves, and able to see at a glance which cubicles were taken, who was waiting to be seen or awaiting treatment. Some patients were waiting for review or transfer.

At first it had daunted Sorcha. Everything was on a far bigger scale than at the small unit she was used to working in. She'd stared at the whiteboard in the same way she'd attempted to read the map of the underground. She was still dreadful at that, but she could now make a decent attempt at the whiteboard.

Certainly she wasn't as expert as May, who must surely have a second degree in logistics, because as Sorcha checked the drugs in the resus trolley, along with Teghan, one of the day staff, May was already armed with a marker and an eraser.

She wrote in the name of the SHO who was the junior doctor on duty tonight—Vanessa.

'And Mr Field's on,' she said. Though her smile didn't last very long. 'Who's the registrar?' she called out, for anyone to answer.

'They're trying to find someone,' Teghan responded from over her shoulder, and then added quietly, for Sorcha's ears only, 'Wait for it! May's going to go off...'

'Find someone?' May squawked, and Sorcha couldn't help but smile as May predictably exploded. 'Are you telling me that I don't have a registrar? How, in the name of all that's holy, are we supposed to cover a trauma team? Every blasted

weekend. No doubt they'll send someone who doesn't know his—'

'It's a pleasure to see you too, May!'

The smile froze on Sorcha's face at the sound of the dry greeting, delivered in a well-schooled voice which every fibre of her being recognised even while her mind fought for it to be otherwise.

It could not be him!

'Oh, Richard, it's you.' May sounded instantly mollified. 'Thank goodness for that, at least.'

Sorcha dared not turn around.

Quite simply, she could not face him.

Not now.

Not here.

Never.

'Morphine sulphate ten mg,' Teghan said, opening up the boxes so that together they could count the ampoules, and Sorcha forced herself to concentrate.

Somehow she got through the rest of the drug check and signed her name. Thankfully his back was to her as she made her way over. He wore black scrubs, and his arms were folded as he was taken through the board by May.

'There you are,' May said, glancing over as Sorcha approached. 'Can I ask you to go to the obs ward first? I know you want to get stuck in.'

'That's fine,' Sorcha responded quickly, more than grateful for the excuse to hide, and fervently hoping that Richard was too busy looking at the patient info and being updated to notice her.

Unfortunately, there was no reprieve.

He turned then, and she was back in the path of his gaze.

It wasn't so warm as the last time their eyes had met, but just for a slip of a second she was back there...lying with him in bed.

Hurriedly, she looked away.

Richard had had a little more warning than Sorcha—albeit a minute at best. But he would never not recognise that hair.

It wasn't just the unique blend of coppers and burnt oranges, but the curl pattern too... And even though her back had been to him, the way it was piled on her head, and the ringlets that danced on her pale, slender neck were familiar.

Weeks on from that night, and seeing her dressed in faded, baggy scrubs, somehow he still recognised the feminine shape beneath. His body certainly did, and he took a breath, pushing out the sight before his eyes, dousing the physical reaction as he recalled the next morning after that night...

That night...

He'd never been able to envisage another relationship. The agony he'd been through was something he could not bear to repeat. For the past three years he'd been treading water just to survive.

Once, for a few moments, he'd briefly looked up, had almost envisaged walking out of that bathroom and telling Sorcha about Jess, but even then he hadn't really been thinking ahead.

Coming out of the bathroom to find her gone...

The only conclusion he'd been able to come to was that she hadn't booked a hotel after all and had only stayed with him because she'd needed somewhere to stay.

It didn't make sense—but then nothing about their night did.

But this was work, and he wasn't going to let things slip here. Richard knew he had to set the tone, so he greeted her straight away.

'Good evening, Sorcha.'

May did a double take. 'You two know each other?'

'Yes,' Richard said.

Sorcha had heard that 'no' could be a complete sentence. She'd never considered it could also be applied to 'yes' but, having given her a brief nod, confirming they knew each other, he offered no more information to May, and neither did she seek it.

'So, Sorcha, can I ask you to take over in the obs ward?'

'Sure.'

It was a relief to escape and head round to the eight-bedded ward used for the consultant's patients. There were only three patients, but it filled quickly, and Sorcha took the handover, which consisted of two head injuries and a gentleman wating for IV antibiotics.

'You've another patient coming in,' the day nurse told her, and Sorcha was relieved when the doors swished open and the new patient arrived.

She was pleased to be busy with an admission.

There certainly wasn't time to examine her thoughts, and near the end of her stint, when Richard appeared on the obs ward, Sorcha didn't know how to address things.

'You have some charts for me?' he said.

'Just some IV antibiotics,' Sorcha responded, completely unable to look at him and glad of the dim light. 'I think the others can wait.'

'Do they need updating or not?' Richard asked.

'Yes,' she croaked, wishing she could be as polite and detached as him, and wishing his scent didn't have all her senses jumping in recall, like little echoes of their time together. She recalled in intimate detail how it felt to lean on his chest, how it felt to breathe in the cologne on his neck…

She hated him. And hated even more how impossibly attractive she still found him. Her hands were shaking a little as she passed him the IV and drug charts to update, though they didn't shake with nerves, more with anger at herself.

'May thinks we know each other.'

'We do.'

She made a soft scoffing noise, then added, 'You could have been more discreet.'

'We helped a collapsed patient at Kings Cross,' Richard said. 'I was never going to go into any more detail.' He carried on writing and then paused. 'I'll need the desk.'

She frowned, and then realised what he meant. There was a chair at one side, but to sit and write at any length he'd need somewhere to put his rather long legs.

'Of course.' She stood. 'I was going to get a cup of tea.' She just wanted to escape, but attempted to be polite. 'Do you want one?'

'No, thank you.'

She didn't go and get a cup of tea as the phone rang then, and it was either lean over him to answer or take a seat on the chair by the desk.

'He's comfortable,' Sorcha told the relative who was calling, and gave updates as Richard worked away. He was making light work of those charts… hopefully by the end of the phone call he'd be gone. 'He'll be reviewed in the morning,' she said. 'If you'd like to ring at about nine?'

Richard wasn't finished. Instead he had taken out the *British National Formulary*—the bible for all medications—and was checking a drug, and Sorcha had to know if this was going to be a regular occurrence.

'I thought you worked in central London?'

'I do,' he responded. 'As well as here.'

'Often?'

'Depends.'

Sorcha swallowed. She'd been hoping—or rather praying—that this was a rare one-off.

'I wasn't expecting to see you.'

'Again,' he said, and looked over.

Sorcha frowned, unsure as to quite what he meant—that little addition sounded as if he'd been finishing off her sentence.

'You didn't expect to see me *again*.'

'I hoped never to,' she admitted.

'I rather guessed that when you fled.' He gave her a thin smile then got back to writing. 'Sorry to disappoint.'

'Excuse me—' Sorcha said, because he'd made it sound as if he was the wronged party.

But there was no chance of continuing because May came through the doors just then.

'Sorcha.' She came over. 'I want to talk to you before I finalise the Christmas off duty. Now, you're working…but I am going to try and give you an early Christmas Day, and I'll see what I can do for New Year's,' May said. 'Can you get home?'

'No,' Sorcha said. 'Besides, my parents are away for New Year.'

'What about you, Richard? Are you in Wales for Christmas?'

'Yes.'

'And how is Jess?'

'Fine,' said Richard, and added his signature to the unfinished notes.

Then he looked over to Sorcha—or rather felt the blast of heat from her cheeks. And when he looked up the flash of anger in her eyes told him she knew about Jess.

How?

'Give her my love,' May said.

'I will. Thanks.'

As May headed off Richard remained, though he certainly wasn't going to discuss such personal matters here.

'We'll speak about this after work; there's a café around the corner,' he said.

'I'm not meeting you.' Sorcha didn't so much as look over at him. 'I've got nothing to say to you.'

'Eight o'clock.' He ignored her protest and named a place she'd never heard of. 'If we're going to be working together then we need to clear the air.'

Not a chance.

There was no way she was meeting him.

And there was no way she could carry on working here.

Somehow, she limped through the night, managing to cross paths with him only occasionally. She even put her hand up to volunteer to take patients up to the ward—usually it wasn't a favourite job, but tonight Sorcha happily obliged.

But at four in the morning there could be no avoiding him.

All the trauma pagers were going off and May was calling her to Resus, so she gowned up.

'What do we know?' Richard asked, already gowned and pulling on gloves as he took the head of the resuscitation bed.

May told him the little she'd been told. It sounded very serious indeed.

'Pedestrian versus car—GCS Three…'

Everyone was given roles, and wore stickers to clearly state who they were. Sorcha was monitor nurse, responsible for undressing the patient and attaching monitors, amongst other things.

'Where's Mr Field?' asked Richard.

'With the aneurism…' said another member of the team.

'Okay,' May said. 'Perhaps, Sorcha, you should be the runner?'

'Sorcha shall be fine as monitor,' Richard said calmly.

Did May think she was too inexperienced?

Sorcha wondered, but there really wasn't time to think it through as visible through the windows was a flash of red and blue lights and soon the paramedics were swiftly entering.

'Male, query in his forties or fifties,' the treating paramedic said. 'Pedestrian versus car. The driver—the only witness—reports he's been unconscious since impact. GCS Three throughout.'

All this was conveyed as the patient was moved from the stretcher, and from there Sorcha got to work. His jumper had already been cut open, so she swapped over the monitors then set to work on his heavy coat.

There was a smell to it that was familiar, and as she sheared through the thick wool she caught the scent of her father coming home.

Richard was assessing the man, and obs were being relayed. 'I want to turn him...'

The patient was desperately injured. His GCS—Glasgow Coma Scale—was the lowest possible, though he was still breathing.

'Any ID?' May asked.

But there was none.

'He's in his pyjamas,' May commented as they cut off his trousers. 'Do you think he was confused and went wandering?'

Richard didn't answer. He was performing a full trauma screen, and as the patient was rolled he checked his back and for anything missed.

'Query closed head injury,' Richard said at last. 'Let's get Neuro down. CT knows to expect him?' he checked.

'They're ready for him,' May said.

'His respiratory rate is decreasing.'

Richard took the decision to intubate before moving him around, and it was swiftly done.

'Let's elevate the head of the bed to thirty degrees,' he said. 'And why are we doing that?'

Sorcha didn't answer. She knew it was to decrease intracranial pressure, but she wasn't going to put up her hand.

'Sorcha?' May prompted, and she had to answer.

'Correct,' Richard said.

He didn't single her out. He just explained things along the way and asked questions—and really he was a very good teacher, reminding everyone of the importance of maintaining the patient's BP between parameters.

The police had arrived, but they'd gleaned little more information.

'Why would he be out at four in the morning?' May wondered aloud.

Sorcha spoke up. 'I think he might be a baker.'

'What?' May said.

'His coat…' Sorcha had caught the sweet doughy scent of it as it had been cut off. 'My father's a baker, and his coat smells like that, and those aren't pyjamas—they look like the twill trousers he wears.'

'A baker?' May said, and one of the policemen chimed in.

'That fits the location, and explains what he'd be doing up so early. The poor guy was probably walking to work.'

The information helped, because in a few moments a car was being sent to a location near the scene of the accident, and by the time they were getting him ready to go to CT they had a possible name.

'There's a Geoff Billings who works there. He didn't turn up for his shift this morning and he's usually early. We're sending a car to his house to check.'

'Well done!' May clucked. 'I would never have got that. What are you, Sorcha? A "super-sniffer"?'

'I must be.' She smiled.

But no, she'd know that scent anywhere—and it brought a lump to her throat to think that this man could be her father, just walking to work, with a coat over his uniform and no ID.

'Where's Neuro?' May asked.

'I'm meeting them in CT,' Richard responded. 'Let's get him round now.'

'Well, why don't I come with you?' May asked, and added, 'Sorcha…if you want to clean up—?'

'May,' Richard interrupted, and then rather sharply added, 'We're fine.'

He briefed the member of staff who would be going to CT. 'Marcus, have five mg of Midazolam ready for any seizure activity.'

Sorcha's cheeks were on fire. Not because of the gowns and PPE, more that May clearly didn't think she was up to taking him.

Still, soon they were in the CT room and getting the patient ready for imaging. Sorcha ensured Mr Billings was covered in the warmer, and helped transfer the equipment, and then they all moved into the pod, closing the door and standing behind a glass screen.

'Richard.' The neuro consultant came in.

'Rafi…'

'I didn't know you were here tonight.'

'I didn't know either,' Richard said.

With greetings over they discussed the patient, but the conversation fell quiet for a long moment as very soon the images came up on the screen.

'Oh, no…' Rafi said, and there were a couple of audible groans. The scans really were dreadful.

The pod fell quiet again.

'Massive midline shift,' Rafi said, then moved to a second screen and scrolled back as the investigation continued.

It was dreadfully sombre, and as the neuro

team discussed their findings it was clear that surgery wasn't an option.

May came in then, and Richard spoke. 'He's suffered a catastrophic head injury,' he said.

May looked at the images for a silent moment. 'Poor man.'

'Yes.'

'I have his wife in the family room,' she said. 'Sorcha was correct. He's a local baker, on his way to work…evidently he just stepped out without looking.'

'I'll come and speak to her now.' Rafi nodded. 'Can we please bring him back to Resus and I'll arrange a bed on ICU?'

'Of course,' May said.

'Keep that blood pressure low, and get his head up to thirty degrees as soon as he's out. What is his wife's name, please?'

'Susan.'

'Is she alone?'

'She's waiting to speak with a doctor before she calls her son.'

They brought him back to the department and into Resus, and May allocated Sorcha to care for him one on one. There was a lot to take care of. Geoff was critically ill and ventilated, so was being continually monitored, and Rafi wanted his blood pressure lower than the usual parameters.

'I'll help tidy him up a bit,' said Jane, wheeling in a trolley with a bowl of water and some toiletries.

'I'm just going to clean your face, Geoff...'

Whether or not he could hear her, Sorcha explained what she was doing, wiping off as much blood and dirt as she could before changing him into a fresh grown.

And perhaps just in time, because May popped her head in then. 'Are there any of the neuro team here?'

Sorcha shook her head. 'I thought Rafi was with you.'

'No.' May came over. 'He spoke to Mrs Billings but then had to head up to ICU.'

She took a breath. Her face was flushed and Sorcha knew she was upset.

'How is she?'

'Confused. I need someone to speak to her again.' She pulled Sorcha aside and spoke in low tones. 'The son's on holiday in France, and his mum has just told him his father's going to be fine and not to come...'

'Problem?' It was Richard.

'Not at all,' May said.

Sorcha frowned—because hadn't May just said otherwise?

'Rafi had to go up to ICU, and May needs someone to speak with Mrs Billings again.'

'I can do that,' Richard said.

'You don't have to, Richard,' May countered. 'I might see if Mr Field is available.'

'May, it's fine,' he said.

He stalked off and Sorcha saw May's lips purse.

'I was hoping to avoid that,' she muttered, and rolled her eyes. 'I'll go in with him.' She went over to Mr Billings and squeezed his hand. 'Your wife will be with you soon, pet.'

Why didn't May want Richard to speak with the wife? Was he too brusque, perhaps?

Sorcha pondered that briefly, though really she was focussed on taking care of Mr Billings. His blood pressure, which had to stay between those strict parameters, kept soaring.

As she checked the drug regime, she could hear loud sobs and shouts, and then a long stretch of silence.

'How is he?' May asked as she came behind the screen, even redder in the face than before. 'He looks very...'

Her mouth wavered, and Sorcha guessed that even close to forty years in the job didn't make you immune from the shock of something like this.

'You've done a nice job.'

Sorcha had found a comb, and also covered up some of the abrasions and cleaned the patient's hands, which were outside the blanket.

'I'll go now and get Susan.'

Only Richard was already bringing in the wife. 'She wants to see him.'

'Of course,' May said.

'Oh, no!' Mrs Billings sobbed when she saw her husband, and May went over and guided her closer. 'Oh, Geoff...'

Sorcha found her a seat, but for now Mrs Billings stood as Richard spoke to her.

'I'll go and ring your son for you, shall I?'

'Please...' She nodded, and when Richard had gone she finally took a seat and held her husband's hand. 'You were supposed to be at work...'

Apart from a quick loo and coffee break, Sorcha stayed with Mr Billings until the day staff took over.

It was a relief when her shift was over, and she changed back into the clothes she'd arrived in, wrapping her scarf round her neck and heading out.

She saw Richard was at the X-ray finder, and she wanted to turn and walk in the opposite direction—but that would look childish.

'I'll see you at eight,' he reminded her as she went past.

'You won't.'

'You're the one who disappeared without a word, Sorcha. You're the one who ran off without explanation.'

'Why do you think that might have been, Richard?'

'Enlighten me.'

'I found out you were married.'

She walked off—marched off, really—out through the black folding doors and into the corridor, still wet from people bringing in the rain from outside. But even if it was pouring it was a relief to be outside and away from him.

'Sorcha...'

She started at the sound of her name, honestly surprised that he'd followed her out.

'Clearly we do need to talk.'

'Clearly we don't!' Sorcha retorted angrily, but Richard would not relent.

'Look, I'd rather have this conversation away from here. I have no idea how you found out I was married, but believe it or not that morning I was about to tell you.'

'Oh, please...' She was angry with him and ashamed of herself. 'What else were you going to tell me? That your wife doesn't understand you? Or that you have an open marriage?' She felt ill—especially now she knew his wife's name, thanks to May's inadvertent slip. 'How *is* Jess?' she sneered.

'In a coma,' Richard responded. 'She has been for the past three years.'

Sorcha didn't react. She didn't say anything at

first—just stared in horror, hating her own poisonous words, so stunned she couldn't think further than that.

'I'll speak to you at eight unless I have to stay back.' He went to walk off, but at the last minute turned. 'I do owe you an explanation but it's a one-time offer, Sorcha—not an open invitation. I try not to bring my private life to work.'

She found her voice then, albeit shaky. 'Or the bedroom?'

Touché, Sorcha thought as she walked off.

But it just didn't feel like a win.

CHAPTER SEVEN

For close to two months, since Richard had come out of the bathroom to find her gone, his thoughts had turned dark when he'd thought about Sorcha.

Now, though, she'd blazed back into his orbit in gorgeous Technicolor—yet the fact there had been a misunderstanding didn't make things easier.

He couldn't allow it to.

Life had already been difficult enough when they'd first met.

It was hellishly complicated now.

He walked in the rain, relieved to be out of the department even while not relishing the thought of sitting opposite Sorcha again.

Or rather, facing the feelings she still evoked.

He pushed open the café door and saw her straight away. She sat twirling a straw in apple juice, and her eyes were wary as he took off his coat and took a seat.

The waitress came over and he ordered a coffee. 'Are you eating?' he asked Sorcha.

'No, thank you,' Sorcha said quickly, clearly wanting this difficult conversation over and done with.

'Just coffee for me, then,' he said, and when the waitress had gone he got straight to it. 'Jess, my wife, is in a care home in Wales.'

'I apologise for what I said before.'

He nodded. 'How did you find out I was married?' he asked. 'Did you go through my wallet?' It was all he'd been able to come up with.

'Not at first,' Sorcha said. 'There was a phone call, on the hotel room phone, and stupidly I answered it. I thought it was about breakfast. But it was somebody looking for you regarding your wife.'

'On the hotel room phone? Why would they…?'

His voice trailed off and he closed his eyes. He swallowed, then his head went back and he sat there for a few seconds.

Then he opened his eyes and met hers.

'I didn't know that they'd tried to reach me at the hotel…' He knew he was making little sense, but the waitress was back, placing down his coffee, and he was glad of the moment to look back. 'I gave them all my contact details—I knew the phones would be off at the conference.' He shook his head. 'They should have called my mobile first.'

'You rang to enquire about Edward,' Sorcha reminded him. 'Maybe the line was busy...'

'It must have been.' He took a deep breath, then pushed on. 'That morning...' He saw a dull blush darken her cheeks and knew she understood the morning to which he referred. 'Jess had taken a turn for the worse, and as it turned out she had pneumonia.'

'What happened to her?' Sorcha asked. 'Did she have a car accident?'

'A horse-riding accident. She suffered severe head and chest injuries.' Her eyes held his and he could see the demand for more information. 'As I said, it's been three years now.'

'It was quite a big thing to miss out while we were talking.'

He gave a wry laugh and saw her look slightly startled. 'I never get to miss it out, Sorcha.'

'I don't understand...'

'You saw how May was last night—and Rafi. Everyone knows, and everyone tries...'

Sorcha looked back on last night with more knowing now. Even though she hadn't noticed anything with Rafi, May had been like a cat on hot bricks around Mr Billings. Or rather, as she now understood, around Richard.

'I was worried May thought I was incompetent.'

'No, that was just May trying to protect me. Look I didn't set out not to tell you…' He called over to the waitress. 'I'm going to get a croissant. You want anything?'

'No, thank you.'

He ordered an almond one, and then carried on speaking. 'I know I messed up, but I wasn't sitting there at Kings Cross, or in the pub, thinking we were going to end up in bed. I was enjoying talking to you—and God knows that's rare these days. Believe me, had I told you, things would have become…'

'Honest?' She finished his sentence for him, but he shook his head.

'I was more honest with you that night than I have been in a very long time.'

She frowned, not understanding what he meant.

'Family, friends…they've been wonderful—I mean that. It's just…' He ran a hand across his brow. 'I honestly don't know where to start.'

His croissant arrived and he dipped it in his coffee.

She asked him a question. 'Why is Jess in Wales?'

'Because…' He shook his head, as if he wasn't going to answer, but then relented. 'Jess lived in Wales and I lived in London.'

'So, you were separated?'

'No.' He gave her a thin smile. 'We've been together since medical school. From the start Jess wanted to be a GP back in Wales and I wanted to work in A&E in London.'

Sorcha felt her own frown.

'We could never pin down where we were going to live and who was going to make the move. We were on holiday once, and realised that was the only thing stopping us from marrying. On everything else we were on the same page. So we decided to make it official and just...'

'Live apart?'

'We didn't see it that way,' he told her. 'Couples commute all the time.'

'I guess...' She thought about it. 'My uncle works on the oil rigs—he's away for ages at a time.'

He smiled at her attempt to understand. 'Well, it's not quite the same. We saw each other all the time, and always made sure our rosters aligned. But we both got to focus on work and we were studying hard too. It might sound unconventional, but it worked for us.'

'You were happy?'

'Very.'

'And you got together at medical school?'

'First term,' he said, and Sorcha felt her eyes widen.

'You were together since you were both eighteen?'

* * *

Richard nodded. 'We got engaged when we were twenty-five and married at thirty.'

'Would you have moved?' Sorcha asked.

'I guess at some point one of us would have.'

'If you'd had a baby?'

'Oh, no.' His response was automatic—the same one he had always given, even before the accident when people had asked about babies. 'Neither of us wanted children.' Richard hesitated, then looked up into the green eyes that had asked him to be honest. 'There was a bit more to it than that, but that's the line we went with.'

'Okay.'

He liked it that she didn't push to know what 'a bit more' meant, just nodded and accepted that there were things he might prefer not to share about his marriage.

'Usually we'd have been together on our days off, but I was about to take the final exam towards my FRCEM when it happened.' Regret flashed across his features and there was a husk in his voice. 'A dog startled her horse.' He put up a hand. 'You don't need to hear all this, but...'

'I'd like to.'

He'd wanted to come straight in, explain as little as possible, and then get out. But he'd completely forgotten how easily they spoke together and the pleasure of sharing conversation with Sorcha.

'I've never told anyone about it from the start,' he admitted. 'Well, apart from medical personnel, of course. But I guess everyone else has lived it with us.'

'Lived it?'

'When the accident first happened and Jess was in ICU people were calling all the time. I ended up sending out group messages. Now I have a group chat for my family, as well as one for Jess's, and another for close friends.'

'Who do you really talk to, though?' Sorcha asked.

'Everyone's been great,' Richard said. 'The thing is…'

She waited.

'They love her too.'

'So you're protecting them?'

'I don't know. I'm probably protecting Jess. She'd hate certain things being discussed. As well as that, I think grief is difficult enough. But because she's still alive… People don't know what to say. Or they say too much.'

'Such as?'

'There are some who suggest I focus on my career, or start dating again. Then there are some who think I should hold out hope, like I did in the beginning.'

He went back to the beginning.

'Jess was in ICU for six weeks, and then for the first year she was MCS.' He realised he was perhaps a little too used to shorthand and said, 'In a minimally conscious state. I was hopeful, though—we all were. Pretty much from the start I knew we weren't going to get her fully back, but Rafi put me on to a rehabilitation place in Europe. I was going to sell my apartment to fund it...we were all on board.'

'All?'

'Her family. She's very close with her parents, and so am I. But then she had a massive bleed. It wiped out all hope—at least it did for me.'

'Not for her parents?'

'No. They clung on, insisted she still had a chance. But...' He shook his head. 'Jess can't regulate her body temperature, so it's hard to know when there's an infection. And that morning, as I said, it turned out she'd developed pneumonia. Trefor, her father, insisted on calling an ambulance, and there was a full resuscitation.'

He watched as Sorcha went to take sip of her drink, clearly not knowing what to say, but her glass was empty.

'With Jess, it's never been as clear cut as with our patient last night. I've tried to maintain shared decision-making—I love her parents. And yet I love Jess more...or loved her. I know she wouldn't have wanted that. Fortunately, we're in agreement now, so we won't put her through that again.'

'I'm so sorry.'

'Thank you.'

'Did you complete your studies?' she asked.

'No.' He shook his head. 'That shiny career that seemed so important back then has been very much put on hold since the accident.'

'Do you miss it?'

It was a question he'd been asking himself, and she looked at him with green eyes that expected an answer.

'At times,' he admitted. 'I still work, but it's not the same being a locum, and I haven't progressed. I'm in Wales a lot—I work there too. And when I come to London, to be honest, it feels like a break.'

'Well, I'm glad you had that little holiday.'

Richard heard the implication and knew she'd decided he'd been looking for a one-night stand.

'It wasn't like that, Sorcha.'

'What was it like, then?' she asked.

'I don't know,' he admitted. 'But it feels like a very long time ago. How are you?' he asked.

'I've wondered.'

Sorcha nodded. 'I've wondered about you, too.'

Despite herself, even while trying hard not

to, she had wondered about him on so many occasions.

The waitress was back and Richard asked for another coffee, and another almond croissant. He glanced at her empty apple juice glass.

'Do you want another?'

She was about to decline, but she did want to speak more rather than dash off, so she nodded. 'But actually…' she looked at the waitress '…I'll have an almond croissant and a tea, please.' She glanced at the selection. 'I'll have a mint tea.'

'What happened to white coffee?'

'If I have one now I'll never get to sleep. I have loud flatmates.' She told him another truth. 'I'm not used to sharing a house. They're probably perfectly lovely—but none of them do shift work and…' She halted, not wanting to be petty about how they pinched her food, the noise, and all the other inconveniences of sharing with strangers. 'Actually, they're awful.'

'That's no good.'

'I'll get through this block of nights and then I'll have to sort something else out.'

'How are things going with Amanda?'

She was touched that he remembered, and also that he asked. 'Not great,' she admitted. 'Still, I'm hoping we can have some time together at Christmas—if May ever finishes the off-duty.'

'How did your parents take the news that you were moving here?'

'They still think I have a mystery man.'

He gave a soft laugh. 'I do have my uses, then?'

'Oh, yes!' She smiled, but it wavered. 'I think they know why I'm really here. To be honest, I wish I'd never come.'

'Really?'

'The flat's dreadful, Amanda's barely home, and—' She looked across the table at him, the latest problem to present itself to her. 'I'm glad we've cleared things up, but...'

He remained a problem.

Now she was no longer hating him, furious at him, she was remembering again just how wonderful their time together had been. How happy and thrilled and content she'd been, all at the very same time.

Now her anger was abating she was somewhat daunted to look into her heart and see the feelings that remained. Those dewy Richard glasses were back on, and she ached to reach for his hand, as she had the morning they'd parted. His jaw was as rough and stubbled as it had been when they'd lain together, and his eyes were still as blue as a northern night.

Their croissants arrived and she took a bite. Instantly she pulled a face. 'That's awful!' The poor waitress glanced over and Sorcha pushed out a smile. 'You have it,' she told him.

'I'm fine.'

'I don't think I can work with you,' Sorcha admitted abruptly. 'I'll work through Christmas, but after that…' She shrugged. 'My friend's only in my flat back in Scotland till the end of January.'

'You're surely not leaving London because of me?'

'Because of a lot of things.'

'You're being ridiculous.'

'I know my limits.'

'Sorcha, things were already complicated when we met. They're hellish worse now. I won't be suggesting we go out to dinner, or fall into bed, or anything else of the sort.'

'I never suggested you would be. But I can't work alongside someone I've slept with.'

'If everyone thought that half the hospital would have to resign!'

'Maybe, but…'

It had come as a shock to find herself still so attracted to him. To sit opposite him again. To look at his pale skin and the shadow on his jaw and to recall how beautiful he looked in the morning.

'Nothing's going to happen,' Richard said. 'I don't know if I've made things clear, but I can't see Jess getting through this. It could be weeks, months...even years. But now that the decision has been made, I'm going to be there for her.'

'As you should be.' Sorcha nodded. 'But I'm far too insecure to be an occasional lover.'

The depths of her own feelings scared her. She'd glimpsed how much losing him had hurt... to fall further for Richard could prove devastating.

'I'm sorry for all you're going through,' she said. And then without thinking, as naturally as breathing, she reached her hand across the table and touched his. 'And for all that's to come.'

His fingers closed around her own, just lightly, and if it was anyone else she thought she would barely have noticed...would simply have taken her hand back. Except she looked down and stared at her own fingers, curling into his, nestling into them like little purring kittens, nudging to be stroked.

And he reciprocated—or rather he didn't let go.

'I can't be your stop gap,' Sorcha said.

'It was never like that.'

'Yes, it was.' Sorcha was being firm—more so with herself. He still held her one hand between both of his now. His hands were cold, but those fingers were still so beautiful, and she knew she should not prolong this conversation. 'You're about to lose the love of your life and—'

'Please don't,' he interrupted. 'I've got enough

people telling me how I should feel and how I should be.'

Sorcha blinked.

'I lost Jess three years ago.'

She looked up then.

'I can tell you the moment I knew she'd gone.'

And now she knew she wasn't getting the amended version, or the group chat version, or anything other than Richard's truth.

'Not here,' Richard said.

And she knew it was not just because half the hospital frequented the café, but more because he could not sit in a public place and voice thoughts that had been kept so long in lockdown.

They walked out into the misty rain and found a little park with gloomy ducks who were huddled under a tree.

'You should have brought your croissant,' Richard said.

'It's bad for them.' Sorcha sighed. 'And it was a bit sickly.' She could still taste the almond. 'It tasted like wedding cake.' She halted. 'Gosh!'

'Stop.' He laughed. 'Please don't be another person who's scared to say the wrong thing.'

'Okay.' She still inwardly winced, but then took a breath and turned and looked at a man she found very beautiful and whose side she didn't want to leave yet.

'How did you know Jess was gone? Was it the scan?'

'I saw the scan, but even then I thought...' He gave a hollow laugh. 'Even then I was still able to override my thoughts. But the neurosurgeon was pretty blunt, and Rafi went through everything for me.'

He sighed, and Sorcha didn't care if it wasn't sensible—she reached over and was soon back holding his hand, telling herself she'd done the same with Mrs Billings, while knowing that it wasn't even close to the same thing.

'It was a couple of weeks later. Trefor was thrilled that she was breathing alone and that her eyes were open, so he and Jess's mother Bronwyn went back home. I think it was the first time I'd been on my own with her since the bleed. Well, I just broke down...'

Sorcha squeezed his hand. Of course she did.

'She didn't react,' Richard said, and he squeezed her hand back. 'Nothing. In fairness, I don't think Jess had ever seen me cry, but...'

Sorcha turned on the bench and looked at him, and she understood now that that had been the moment he'd known.

'There was nothing,' he said again. 'I knew she was gone.'

'And you haven't told anyone?'

'Not really. It feels disloyal.' He looked back at

her. 'Do you remember saying you felt like that about your parents?'

'Yes.'

'Well, it's much the same. It's something I've dealt with. How I felt privately didn't change things. I've been working through it, and I'm getting there—albeit slowly. That afternoon, when the trains were cancelled, I was relieved not to have to go.'

He took a breath, as if surprised he'd admitted it out loud.

'I'm never going to divorce her, or stop visiting her, but I think that day I knew I was ready to join the human race again. Things have changed now, though.'

'I get that.'

'I'm mainly based in Wales.'

'You've still got a house in Wales?'

'No.' He shook his head. 'I knew she was never coming back to it, and we had to sell it to pay for her care. I don't think Trefor's forgiven me for that, but it was that or sell my apartment here.'

'You would have sold it for her rehab, though?'

'In a flash,' Richard said. 'But that was when I had hope. I didn't live at the house much when she was alive, but it was hell being there without her. I couldn't live there just to appease her parents.'

'No,' Sorcha agreed.

'Do you still wish I'd told you all this?'

'Of course,' Sorcha said, and then halted. 'I don't know,' she admitted. 'If you had I think we'd have spent the night talking rather than...'

Sorcha blushed and let out a small laugh. How he'd missed that sound. And even on this bleak, grey morning the light, breathy sound brought a reaction, for his lips moved into a soft smile.

'I think that night was perfect just as it was,' Sorcha told him. 'Except for that phone call the next morning.'

'Yes, and except for me coming out to find you gone.' He looked at her lips, tinged blue with the cold, and then up to her eyes. 'I didn't mean to hurt you.'

'I know that now.'

'You're okay?'

'Apart from freezing,' she admitted, and together they stood.

He'd been through so much, thought Sorcha, and she was sure he had a lot more to come. She believed he thought he'd grieved his wife, but it wasn't as straightforward as that.

There was no end in sight and his ties to Jess's family were still strong.

And she liked him far too much.

'How often do you work at The Primary?' she asked as they walked towards the park gates.

'It varies,' he said. 'I've got a shift next week and a couple the week after. It really all depends. Sorcha, please don't think about leaving on my account.'

'It's not just you,' she admitted. 'I haven't really been happy since...' She stopped then, unsure if the blues she'd felt lately had started when she'd arrived in London or when she'd found out about Jess.

Since that night the world hadn't felt the same.

'I think we go our separate ways here,' she said. 'My flat's back that way. Are you getting the Tube?'

'I am.'

It was, Sorcha found, very hard to say goodbye.

After a night wondering how she could avoid him, now she didn't know how to tear herself away.

'Bye,' she said, a little too quickly, and turned and walked away.

'Sorcha...?'

She turned.

'Is everything okay?'

'I just told you.' She shrugged. 'I'm fine. It's just been...'

He walked towards her. 'I meant we had a contraception fail...'

'And?' She frowned. 'I told you—I'm on the pill.'

'You've gone off coffee...' he said.

'I hate the milk here in London.' Sorcha rolled her eyes. 'Richard, there's nothing to worry about in that department.'

'And the croissant?'

'Richard, I'm fine.'

'You look—' He halted in whatever he'd been about to say.

'Just say it.'

'I hate it when people tell me I've lost weight or I'm looking tired,' he said.

'Go ahead.'

'You've got dark circles under your eyes.'

'I have been working all night.' She chose not to tell him about the many sleepless nights she'd suffered thinking of him. 'Honestly, everything's fine.'

'Good.'

She should turn and walk away. Only if it had been hard enough the first time, it felt near impossible now. And it must be hard for him, too, because suddenly he took her arms and pulled her into him.

'Sorcha...'

'Please don't say sorry.'

'I wasn't about to,' he said.

She listened to the steady thump of his heart and it was the oddest thing... When she should be in turmoil at being back in his arms, it was the calmest and steadiest she'd felt in weeks.

'We should have ended things better,' he told her.

'Yes...'

This felt by far nicer.

And when he lifted her chin so she'd look up at him, it was a much sweeter parting than their last one.

'Your lips are blue...' he said, and then lowered his head to put that right.

He brought her lips to colour and to life, soft and warm, and as their mouths moved slowly she moulded to his body, leant into his warmth.

It was bliss to be kissed by him and to be back in his arms.

Yet what could he offer her?

A day here and there? The odd night.

Or would he ask her to hold on? Because that meant he was waiting for his wife to die before he resumed life.

'Take care,' Richard said.

'And you.'

CHAPTER EIGHT

SORCHA SLEPT THROUGH the days and worked at night, telling herself she didn't miss Richard or want him.

Her final night shift at work was wild. If the department had been busy on her arrival, at midnight it all kicked off—and Sorcha got the big inner city nursing experience she'd hoped for.

Fights and stabbings.

It was a relief not to think of Richard for a while. To be so damn busy that she forgot how much she missed him and how wonderful their brief time together had been.

She was literally running at one point, dashing a patient up to Theatre—a rather famous patient, apparently, not that Sorcha had heard of him.

It was a serious run and she was suddenly all breathless, the lights spinning.

'Are you okay?' the theatre nurse checked.

'Fine.' Sorcha put her head down for a moment. 'I haven't run like that since…' Her mind went back to the moment before Richard had entered her life. Running for the train at Kings Cross. 'Don't mind me.'

To her horror, she found that she was crying.

'Sorcha?' David, one of the porters, came over. 'Whatever's wrong?'

'It's nothing.' She pressed fingers into her eyes. 'I'm just tired.' She waved his concern away. 'You go back. I might go and get a cookie, or something, from the machine.'

It was suitably awful, but sugary and sweet, and Sorcha ate it greedily as she made her weary way back to A&E.

By seven a.m. the sugar rush had long since worn off and Sorcha stood pale and tired and more than ready for bed. Or rather ready to head back to her flat and her noisy, celebratory flatmates, who wouldn't care a jot that she'd been working all night.

She heard May speaking. 'Morning, Mr Field,' she said, greeting the consultant. 'You're early.'

'I'm not.'

'Goodness,' May said. 'Is that really the time? Sorcha, take a marker and help me update the board.'

She read out the names of the medical staff taking over in the morning.

'So, Mr Field…?' Sorcha started.

'When's he retiring?' Jane asked as she cleaned down the trolleys for the morning.

'Not for a while,' May said. 'I think he's here till summer.'

'Who's replacing him?' she asked, but May only shrugged.

'I have no idea.' She got back to reading out names. 'Mr Owen is also on. Hold on…' She sighed. 'No, he's on leave. Maybe Dr Lewis…'

'Might Richard replace Mr Field?' one of the nurses suggested, and Sorcha felt her neck stiffen and her ears prick up to high alert. 'I thought he'd be a consultant by now.'

'He hasn't got his FRCEM,' May said, and Sorcha knew that was the qualification he'd been studying for when the accident had occurred. 'God, but I wish it could be him.'

'He's not exactly fun, though,' Jane said.

'Do you want fun,' May asked, 'or your life saving? Anyway, he's gorgeous. That voice and those blue eyes… If I was thirty years younger…'

'May!' Jane yelped. 'You can't say those things any more.'

'Of course I can. And if I can't, with a bit of luck they'll fire me.'

It was clear that they all adored Richard, and Sorcha could see he wasn't just a casual locum but a part of the fabric here. He worked here when he could…when his complicated life allowed.

And apparently he was working this morning.

Not until nine, though, and she was relieved

that their paths wouldn't cross. She just couldn't pretend to be okay any more.

She'd been so angry with him, but she'd refused to cry over a cheat. Now, since she'd found out about Jess, she felt raw—as if their one night together had occurred just last week. The pain of them being over was as new as if it had happened then.

Perhaps she'd used her anger as a shield?

Now, though, it felt as if that shield was dissolving—as if there was nothing between her and the memory of them together.

'You look dead on your feet,' May commented to her as she brought over the drug trolley keys and then scuttled off to take handover. 'If any journalists call about our famous patient, remember to say no comment.'

'I know.'

'The police are trying to find out about the stabbing. It's an active investigation.'

'I know they are.'

Sorcha sat on a stool at the nurses' station and answered the phone when it rang, but it wasn't a journalist, and she directed the enquiry up to Theatre.

The next call was a relative of their famous patient. Or she said that she was.

'Is he there?' she demanded.

'I'm sorry, I can't give that information out,' Sorcha said.

It was tough, but the patient had requested confidentiality. His parents were both in the waiting room, and they had told the staff that all relevant parties had already been informed.

'Can't you at least tell me if he's there?' the woman asked.

'I'm sorry, I can't give you that information.'

Oh, she ached for it to be seven-thirty.

'Journalist?' Vanessa checked, and Sorcha nodded. 'Can I just have a quick hand?' the junior doctor asked.

'Sure,' Sorcha said, jumping down from the stool.

'I need to take some blood from a patient, but he's a bit cantankerous.'

She followed Vanessa into the cubicle, where there was a large man asleep and snoring.

'Mr Dennis?' Vanessa said, and the man awoke, startled.

'Hello,' Sorcha said, introducing herself. 'The doctor just wants to take another look at you and get some blood.'

As quickly as that, things changed.

Mr Dennis sat bolt upright and struck out at the junior doctor, and as Sorcha called for assistance he jumped down from the gurney.

Sorcha would have run—she was rather good at

that—but her back was to the wall, and the patient was on the other end of the gurney between them.

'Mr Dennis...' She kept her voice calm. Vanessa was leaning on the wall and holding her shoulder, and David was rushing in to assist. Help had arrived.

This sort of scene unfortunately wasn't unfamiliar, but suddenly, for the first time since September, time slowed down.

Sorcha saw Mr Dennis's hands reach for the gurney. 'No!' she said. But it had already moved. She moved to cover her stomach but she was too late. He slammed the gurney straight into her midriff.

The shock was as searing as the pain—and then everything went white.

The scuffle was over, Security was arriving and already Mr Dennis was compliant. Sorcha sat up against the cubicle wall, unsure if she was hurt or even what had taken place.

Everyone was rushing, and poor Vanessa was being led out, still holding her shoulder, as May came over to where Sorcha sat.

'I'm okay,' Sorcha said. 'I think I'm just winded.'

She attempted to stand, but May was having none of it.

'Stay there,' May told her. 'You're as white as a sheet. Sarah?' she called to another colleague. 'I need a gurney right away.'

'Not for me.' Sorcha pushed up on her hands. 'Honestly, I'm fi—' Except she wasn't, and she sank back down and doubled over. 'I can't get my breath…'

'You're okay,' May said, and she was so calm and reassuring that Sorcha was able catch her breath and take a deep one in. Then another. 'That's it…'

'I'm okay…' Sorcha agreed.

'Come on.'

May helped her onto the gurney and soon she was in a cubicle of her own, being helped into a pale lemon gown.

'How are you feeling?' May asked as she covered her with a blanket and checked her obs.

'I'm okay,' Sorcha said again, and nodded. 'I just feel a bit…'

'A bit what?'

'Nauseous,' she admitted.

'You got a fright,' May said. 'Your blood pressure's a bit low. I might just put a line in…'

'I don't need a cannula.'

'I'll tell that to Mr Field, shall I? When he asks why I didn't put one in when your blood pressure's in its boots.' She turned and smiled. 'Here he is now.'

Mr Field gave her a smile, followed by a sigh. 'Hello, Sorcha, I'm so sorry this has happened.'

He was very kind, and asked if there was anything in her medical history he needed to know, but there really wasn't anything.

And then he examined her.

Thoroughly.

'It's just a bruise,' Sorcha grumbled.

'Indeed, you are bruised.' Mr Field nodded. 'And it's over your spleen. I'm not going to take any chances.' He sat her forward and palpated her back, over her kidneys, and asked many of the same questions he already had. 'We'll get a urinalysis to check for blood, and also a BHCG...'

Sorcha had already told him that she wasn't pregnant, but she knew Mr Field was thorough, and wouldn't send her for an abdominal X-ray without one.

She was left alone then. May had nodded when she'd asked for the curtain to be closed, and it was odd to lie there and hear the sounds of A&E without being a part of the action.

She closed her eyes when she heard Richard arrive, and could hear him being brought up to speed by the nursing staff.

Very soon the curtain was swished aside.

'Hey...' Richard came in and closed the curtain behind him. 'I just heard. Are you okay?'

'It's nothing,' she said. 'May insisted I was seen.'

'Of course you had to be seen. What did Mr Field say?'

'Not much.' Sorcha shrugged. She felt teary, and that wasn't like her at all, and she felt dreadfully exposed too. 'I'm to have an abdominal X-ray, and I'm on this stupid drip. I think he's just making a fuss because I'm staff.'

'Mr Field is thorough with everyone,' Richard said. 'And you are rather pale.'

'I'm always pale,' she said.

'I heard that the day we met,' Richard said, 'and you were seconds away from fainting then.'

'I'm always like that.' She actually smiled. 'I mean, if anything happens—even just a lack of sleep. I used to always get out of sports at school…'

'I bet.' He smiled. 'But Mr Field doesn't know you like I…' He halted, and then tried to change the personal recollection into a little joke. 'He doesn't know what a sickly thing you are.'

'Peely-wally,' Sorcha said.

'Pardon?'

'That's what we call it at home.'

'Your parents say that to you?'

'Not just my parents.' She smiled. 'Patients say it, and if you worked up there and didn't know what it meant, after a couple of shifts you would.'

'Seriously?' He smiled. 'What does it mean?'

'Pale and sickly. Off-colour.'

'Well, you're definitely looking peely-wally, then,' he said, and took her hand.

She pulled it back. 'Don't,' she said. 'If anyone comes in they'll think there's something going on between us.'

'Because there *is* something going on,' Richard said, almost angrily. 'Hell, Sorcha—'

His voice broke off as May came in, bearing a bedpan.

This was not the look Sorcha had been hoping for!

'I am not using that.' Sorcha was adamant. 'I can get up.'

Richard smiled as he headed out, leaving May to convince Sorcha she was not to get up.

Then the smile faded.

He felt a little peely-wally himself.

The sight of Sorcha on the trolley, and hearing the news that she was injured…

'Upsetting, isn't it?' Mr Field commented as he joined him at the central station.

'Very,' Richard agreed. 'Where were Security when all this happened?'

'They were in the waiting room and at the main entrance,' Mr Field said. 'They can't be everywhere, Richard.'

Mr Field was always fair—he didn't jump to blame anyone—and Richard was usually the same. But this morning his responses felt less rational. 'What's happening now?' he asked.

'I'm going to send Vanessa to the obs ward for a few hours. It's possibly overkill, but she lives alone.'

Richard was doing his best to focus, and to nod in all the right places, but while he was concerned for Vanessa, right now his exasperation and distress was solely for Sorcha, however unfairly proportioned.

It was personal.

But then Vanessa was a colleague also.

He took a breath and knew it was all about his feelings for Sorcha—that despite attempts to dismiss them, to cut them out, they flourished like some untamed garden.

'Surely we can get Sorcha X-rayed now,' he said, irritated that she was presumably having to wait until nine, when the department officially opened. 'I know it's not technically urgent, but…'

'It's not that,' Mr Field said. 'When I was examining Sorcha…' His voice trailed off as May came over.

She gave Mr Field a nod. 'You were right,' May said. 'I don't think she has so much as a clue.'

Richard frowned.

'I'll go and talk to her now,' Mr Field said, but May shook her head.

'It might be better for her to hear it from me.'

'Hear what?' Richard said, and May looked slightly away.

It was just a tiny flash of avoidance, and had he not known her so well he wouldn't have even noticed it. But he did.

'I'm not going to run around with a megaphone,' Richard said, knowing damn well May was protecting her staff member. But he had this gut feeling... Or was it just the thump of realisation as to why the X-ray was being delayed? The possible findings in the routine urinalysis? The pregnancy test Mr Field *always* insisted on in any female patient of child-bearing age?

'Sorcha's pregnant?' he checked, and May gave a tight nod.

'I could feel her fundus,' Mr Field said. 'Ten to twelve weeks, I'd say. I agree, May.' He nodded now. 'It might be better coming from you.'

'No,' Richard said immediately. 'I'll tell her.'

'It's fine.' Mr Field stood firm. 'I think May can break the news more gently—and anyway, she isn't your patient.'

'Sorcha definitely isn't my patient,' Richard agreed and then added, 'I'll tell her.'

And he really could convey a lot with few words, because Mr Field's eyes widened slightly and May went a little pink, her lips pursed as he made it clear he wasn't going in there as Sorcha's doctor.

And possibly his gulp of air and rapid blink

had them guessing he was more than a colleague or a friend…

Sorcha was pregnant.

And, as sure as eggs were eggs, he knew it was down to him.

He'd never run away from a tricky situation in his life and he wasn't about to start now.

If Sorcha had to find out she was pregnant at work and deal with people knowing, then so too could he.

'I'll tell Sorcha. If you could give us some privacy, please?'

'Of course.' May's face reddened as she nodded.

'When you speak with her,' Mr Field said, 'can you let her know that I'll be asking the surgeons to take a look and, given her status, I'd like the obstetrician to check her over?' He glanced at the time. 'I'll wait for them to change over.'

'Who's on from Obstetrics today?' Richard asked, and May, who was already in the middle of changing the whiteboard, answered quickly.

'Monica,' she said. 'She's excellent.'

'I know.' Richard nodded.

Monica was the colleague who had seen them that night getting into the lift at the hotel—but, more to the point, she was Jess's closest friend.

He didn't have the capacity to think about that

now. He just filed it away as he walked towards the cubicle.

Opening the curtain, he smiled at a rather wan and visibly bored Sorcha, who lay there rolling her eyes as he came in.

'I want to go home,' she said immediately. 'But now I have to wait until X-Ray opens.'

'You're not going for an X-ray.'

'Good,' she said, and moved to sit up.

But the gurney was flat, and it wasn't such an easy manoeuvre—or perhaps her stomach did, in fact, hurt, he thought. Because mid attempt to sit up she lay back down.

'How do you feel?' he asked.

'Stupid,' she admitted. 'I shouldn't have got between the wall and the gurney.'

'It happened,' Richard said. 'There isn't always time to think straight.'

He smiled at the irony of his own words—something had happened that night, and neither of them had been thinking straight then.

'Sorcha, the reason they're not sending you for an X-ray...' He paused, briefly wavering from his usual direct approach, then reminding himself that a long preamble would be both confusing and pointless. 'You're pregnant.'

Her response was immediate. 'No.'

Sorcha's voice was calm, and he looked into

her green eyes to see the slight smile on her lips that told him he was mistaken.

'I'm not.'

'Yes.'

She blinked, and he watched as the possibility started to impinge, a tiny frown forming on her brow. And then she hauled herself from acceptance.

'The test must be wrong.'

'It's not just the test,' Richard responded. 'Mr Field already thought you were—he could feel your fundus when he examined you.'

'Then he's wrong,' Sorcha said, in a voice that was no longer calm—instead it edged on defiance. 'This is ridiculous.'

She again went to sit up, but Richard's hand went to her upper arm and halted her panicked response. So she lay back down, her eyes closing for a moment as she wrestled with the facts he'd so calmly delivered.

'Sorcha, if he can feel the fundus, you're around twelve weeks along.'

'I didn't have sex twelve weeks ago,' she retorted sharply.

'Add two weeks.' Richard smiled unseen at her slight belligerence, but he didn't quite know why. Maybe just because he was watching her argue with herself as she lay there. 'And we *both* know you had sex around ten weeks ago.'

Her eyes opened then and met his. He saw for the first time a flash of tears, and understood that she was completely overwhelmed.

Oh, Sorcha was indeed overwhelmed—completely.

She couldn't be pregnant!

Panic was kicking in now.

And if she was pregnant—*pregnant!*—then shouldn't she be finding out alone, not being informed by the damn father?

She hated it that she was at work, and even if she loathed her poky, unfriendly flat, she'd give anything to be there now to absorb these new facts.

'I want to go home.'

It was always her first instinct.

To run.

She knew she was being ridiculous, and Richard's hand was still on her arm. But even before he could halt her from sitting up, she sank back down.

'It's okay,' Richard said.

'It really isn't,' she retorted, then put her arm over her face, shielding herself, trying to fathom it all. Her hand went down to her stomach...to her still-flat stomach. 'I'd know if I were pregnant.'

'You have gone off coffee,' Richard pointed

out. 'And you are, as May said after your sleuthing with Mr Billings, a super-sniffer.'

From behind the shield of her arm she gave a half-laugh and thought of all the odd little things that had been happening.

'I am tired,' she admitted. 'I thought it was the move, and not getting good-quality sleep in my flat-share. Plus I suppose I've been more upset than usual.'

'About Amanda?'

'Yes,' she said. And then, because she was too confused to lie, admitted— 'And about what happened with you...' She winced as she said it. 'I mean, I should have got over it, of course...'

'I know,' he agreed, and removed his hand. 'I get that, Sorcha.'

He was being very kind, if a little distant. He let her be quiet for quite some considerable time, and she had no idea if it was his professional persona, or if he was shell shocked too. Or perhaps he just didn't know what to say.

It was then that she thought of his situation.

'What about Jess?'

'Maybe don't think about that now?' he suggested. 'Just think about you.'

'No, but...' She was suddenly all fluttery inside. 'My parents. How do I tell them?' She thought of their disappointed faces. 'Pregnant after a one-night stand with a married man. They'll never forgive me!'

'Sorcha...'

'It's true, though. Even if they understand about Jess, it was still just one night...' She lay silent for a moment and then looked up at him. 'Aren't you going to ask?'

'Ask what?'

'If it's yours.'

'I was there that night,' he said, and even if that didn't make perfect sense, she understood what he meant. That night had been so special—of course this baby was his.

Baby!

'An obstetrician's going to come and review you,' Richard said. 'It might be a while. Sorcha...?' She heard slight discomfort in his voice. 'Do you remember that we met a friend of mine that night, when we were coming out of the lift at the hotel? A fellow doctor called Monica?'

She frowned.

'She's on call today, so it will be her. But I can ask for someone else...'

Sorcha put her arm back over her head and lay silent.

May came in. 'Sorcha,' she said, 'Monica's said she'll be down shortly. She has a paramedic with her—he's on professional development—she's asked if you'd mind him accompanying her?'

'That's fine,' Sorcha said—it was a teaching hospital after all. And then she heard Richard speak.

'May, could we perhaps see if...?'

'It's fine,' Sorcha said, before he could ask for another doctor to take over her care. It would make things even more awkward, Sorcha thought, and anyway, everyone would soon know.

In all honesty, if Richard hadn't told her who she was, Sorcha wouldn't have recognised Monica. She was dressed in a dark navy suit, with her long hair tied back, and she didn't recognise Sorcha.

At least not at first.

'Hello.' Monica smiled and introduced herself, as well as the paramedic who was with her. 'This is Luke.'

'Thanks for this,' Luke said.

'Now...' Monica glanced at the notes. 'You've had two shocks this morning.' She smiled at Richard. 'You think she's around twelve weeks?'

'That was Mr Field's assessment,' Richard responded.

And then his voice went a touch thick. Not embarrassed—Sorcha couldn't quite define it—but he took her hand.

'We think that's right,' he said.

He gave her hand a squeeze, and she watched

as Monica did a brief double-take as she realised Sorcha wasn't actually his patient.

Then he looked at Sorcha's red hair and swallowed. 'We had a contraceptive failure at the end of September,' Richard said. 'It must have been then...' He stopped, as if trying to pinpoint things.

With that one statement he'd made them sound as if they were more involved than a one-night fling, and she was grateful for that.

And, when your innards were being served up for several departments in your workplace to pore over, it very much helped to keep some details private. Sorcha gratefully squeezed his hand back.

'Right,' Monica said, back to being steady and efficient after her earlier very brief falter. 'Richard, could you excuse us for just a moment?'

'Of course.'

'Luke, would you mind stepping out, too? Just briefly.'

'Of course.'

'Sorcha,' Monica said when they were alone. 'I'm not sure if you're aware that I'm a friend of Richard...'

'And Jess,' Sorcha added, so that Monica didn't have to.

'Yes.' She nodded. 'I will understand completely if you'd rather I called a colleague to take care of you.'

'It's fine. I don't need someone else.'

'I will have to ask you some quite personal questions,' she warned. 'Not just now—I have to get back to the unit—but I'll be taking a thorough history and I don't want you to think for a moment that you can't speak freely and frankly. Anything you tell me is confidential. I want you to know that.'

'Yes, I understand.'

'I have to ask my patients about mental health… domestic violence and such.'

'We're not living together.'

'Even so…' Monica gave her a smile. 'Sorcha, I'd like to take care of you. I just want to be certain you're okay with that.'

'Yes.'

'And if you change your mind, that's okay too.'

'Thank you.'

While they were alone, Monica asked if this was her first pregnancy—it was—and if there had been any gynaecological problems or procedures in her past, or anything that it would serve her better for Monica to know.

'Nothing…' Sorcha thought back. 'Except I'm on the mini-pill, and I've been taking it all along.'

'That's fine. It's very common and nothing to worry about.' Monica smiled reassuringly. 'Shall I let them back in now?'

'Yes.'

Sorcha admired Monica for pausing the consultation and confronting the situation immediately, and when both men returned she resumed where they'd left off.

'So, a contraceptive fail at the end of September, then.' She explained things to Luke as she went. 'Sorcha's been taking the mini pill. Have you had any pregnancy symptoms, Sorcha?'

'None.'

'She's gone off coffee,' Richard added, and she was grateful for him mentioning that, as it made them almost sound like a couple. Perhaps it shouldn't matter to Sorcha what people thought, only it did.

It mattered to her, and she rather thought it might one day matter to their baby.

'Any morning sickness?' Monica asked.

'None,' Sorcha said. 'Well, perhaps a bit, but nothing I've really noticed.'

'I'm just going to check your blood pressure,' Monica said.

'It's always a bit low,' Sorcha told her.

'It is,' Monica agreed. 'But it's on the low end of normal. Have you eaten this morning?'

'A giant chocolate cookie...' Sorcha recounted her sins. 'A bag of crisps...'

Sorcha turned as May came in. 'And some mint slices,' May reminded her.

'Okay.' Monica nodded. 'Let's have a look at your stomach.'

Sorcha saw Richard's slight grimace at the sight of her abdomen and Monica's eyes briefly flashed. 'You're going to have quite a bruise…' She gently palpated the area where the injury had occurred, again explaining things to Luke. 'The mother's health has to come first. We can't just worry about the baby if she's bleeding elsewhere. I'll be putting in another IV—I think that's wisest. With any blunt trauma in pregnancy it's good to have two lines in.'

She smiled to Sorcha.

'Sorry that I'm talking over you, but I'm talking to Luke about a more advanced pregnancy. Your little one is still quite tucked away.' Monica moved her hands further down. 'Yes…' She called Luke over and he had a feel of her fundus, and then Monica smiled and took Sorcha's hand, placing it gently where her own and Luke's had just been. 'Can you feel that?'

There was a little wedge of muscle just above her pubic bone.

'Yes,' Sorcha nodded. 'Though barely…'

'It's just starting to emerge, but I'd certainly put you at ten to twelve weeks…'

She spoke to Luke for a moment, and Sorcha lay with her eyes closed, wondering how she hadn't known.

'Richard, could I ask you to wait outside again?' Monica asked.

This time Luke stayed, though he remained at the head of the bed as Monica performed a gentle internal.

Again she spoke to Luke. 'You'd ask if there was any bleeding, or if the waters had ruptured… check underwear if the patient's unconscious.' They discussed seat belt injuries as Monica replaced the blanket and then removed her gloves. 'Everything seems fine, Sorcha.'

Sorcha couldn't take it in and she didn't know how she felt—let alone fathom how Richard must be feeling.

'It's a lot,' Monica said. 'I was just explaining to Luke that if you were further along we'd put you on a CTG monitor and observe for a few hours.' Monica paused. 'You've obviously had no prenatal care? We'll get some blood work done, the same as I do for all my prenatal mothers, and we'll do a cross match, just in case. For now, we'll get an ultrasound to check dates and the position of the placenta. And I might ask the surgeons to come and take a look—just to check your spleen. I do tend to err on the side of caution. We'll keep you nil by mouth for now.'

'Can't you check if the baby's okay now?' Sorcha said, suddenly desperate to know that the incident hadn't hurt the little life inside her. 'With a Doppler?'

'Sorcha, its heart will be the size of an apple

pip. I don't want you to get upset with me trying to locate it. It's better that we do an ultrasound and find out what we're dealing with.'

'Okay.'

'I know my colleague Sandra is on this morning. I was just talking to her about another patient. She's excellent. I'll ask her to take care of you, and she'll let me know.' She filled out a mountain of forms. 'Do you know your blood group?'

'I don't,' Sorcha admitted.

'Okay, after the ultrasound—so long at the surgeons are happy—we'll move you up to Antenatal and I'll come and see you there.'

She smiled at Sorcha and she and Luke trooped out, and then Richard came back in.

'It's all okay,' he said.

'It's not, though.' She heard the shudder in her breathing. 'I don't know what to do.'

'Nothing for now,' Richard said. 'We just need to make sure that you're well.'

There was a flurry of activity as the surgeons came and checked her, and then there was a long lull, but finally she was being moved to Imaging.

'What a morning you're having,' May said. 'And from here they're going to take you up to Antenatal.'

There was so much to think about that Sorcha found she couldn't concentrate on one single thing, so she just watched the ceiling whizz by and then waited in a corridor until a porter came and wheeled her towards a radiography room.

'Do you want to come in?' she asked Richard, who really did look a little grey now. 'I'll get it if you don't.'

'I'll come.'

Richard heard his own rather terse tone and moved to check it, although he actually felt a little ill. Not from lack of sleep, or even the events of this morning...just from being in Imaging, with someone he cared about, ready to find out if all was well with the baby he'd only just discovered Sorcha was carrying.

It was different from what had happened with Jess, of course, but it felt somewhat the same. He pushed that worry aside and made small talk with Sandra, the radiographer, as Sorcha slid onto the examination table.

'We're just checking your upper abdomen first, where the apparent injury is...' Sandra said, and Richard knew they were first checking for anything acute that might need urgent attention.

'I didn't think you'd ever be seeing my spleen,' Sorcha said to Richard.

'Nor me.'

He smiled, but it was a forced one. There were simply too many memories raining in as he recalled looking at the mess of Jess's images and standing behind the glass in a closed-off pod.

'Are you okay, Richard?' Sorcha asked worriedly.

She'd obviously picked up on his discomfort, though he was trying very hard to hide it from her.

'Yes,' Richard answered, reminding himself that surely he should be the one asking Sorcha that. 'How do *you* feel?'

'Honestly? Fine. Just nervous.'

'There's no sign of contusion...' said Sandra, and Richard was relieved that there were no signs of bleeding and everything appeared normal. 'Everything looks fine.'

'I meant...'

He knew Sorcha was worried about the baby. Scared to find out that she was pregnant one minute and then wasn't the next.

The radiographer moved the probe lower, and Richard saw that Sorcha was holding her breath.

Then they heard the heartbeat and saw it on the screen...the baby's heartbeat...whooshing and rapidly galloping.

'Goodness,' Richard said, unable to move his eyes from the screen.

There was a whole other world there...a whole life. It was moving, and perfect—a little cord, and legs, tiny feet and a face.

And while he still didn't know how he felt, the images told him what mattered right now.

He'd always tried to be a good man, but he swore to do better.

As they waited for Sorcha to be moved up to Antenatal he had a suggestion. 'Why don't you stay at mine for a while?'

'Yours?' Sorcha shook her head. 'We don't know each other. We're hardly—'

'Just listen for a moment. You need to rest, and at some point we need to talk. Your flat share doesn't sound ideal.'

'No, it isn't. But I feel that I want to be on my own.'

'I can drive you up to your parents', if you'd prefer—?'

'No,' she interrupted. 'I won't get any rest there.' She gave a weak laugh. 'I love them dearly, but this is going to rock their world.'

'It hasn't rocked mine.'

Richard's voice was steady, and the grey tinge had gone from his complexion. Perhaps a man who had already lost so much dealt with things more calmly. Or perhaps... Her mind darted. Perhaps he didn't really care. Perhaps it was an inconvenience?

'We're going to be parents, Sorcha.'

'Yes.'

'So why don't we try to communicate?'

'I'm not brilliant at that.'

'I had noticed.' He smiled.

'And I don't like arguments.'

'Good, because neither do I.' Then, as he held her gaze, he made another suggestion. 'Stay at mine while you recover from this. I'm not going to demand answers, or police your future. You can stay in your room like a moody teenager if you want. But you're not well, and this is *our* child.'

'Living together, though…?'

'Sorcha, I am not asking you to permanently move in.' He hadn't even fully lived with his wife. 'Just think about it…'

She nodded.

'Do you want me to go now?' he asked. 'Give you some space?'

She didn't know the answer to that question. Did she want to be alone to process things? Right now things felt a little better with him here.

'Thank you for being the one to tell me,' Sorcha said. 'How did you find out?'

'May was looking guilty and trying to speak to Mr Field discreetly.' He gave a smile. 'I think she'd guessed we might not have just met the once at Edward's cardiac arrest.'

'How?'

'We like each other, Sorcha.' He was as direct as always. 'Even if we try not to admit it or show it.'

She was silent, unsure how to respond.

'If you do come to mine, nothing will happen. We will have separate rooms—I can assure you of that. We have too much to sort out without confusing things further.'

'Confusing things?'

'We're not a couple. Other people are going to think that we are, but…' His words sort of punched her in the heart with a velvet glove. 'But we *are* going to be parents. It might be nice to know where we're at before we tell the world.'

Sorcha was moved up to Antenatal then, and placed in a little four-bedded ward. She was too tired to think, let alone think straight.

'Perhaps I would like a rest,' she told Richard.

'Okay. Let me know what's happening later.' Then he clicked his tongue. 'I don't even have your phone number.'

It felt ridiculous for her to be pregnant with his baby and he didn't even have that, but Richard was right. They weren't a couple. Still, they exchanged phone numbers.

'I'll go and tidy the flat in case I have a guest arriving.'

Sorcha wasn't so sure about that. While it would give them a chance to talk, and it would certainly be a more conducive place to heal than her flat share, Sorcha wasn't so sure it was the sensible choice.

She liked him.

A lot.

More than she dared admit even to herself.

And she was having his baby.

When he'd gone, a midwife came and told her she was no longer nil by mouth. 'I've got some sandwiches for you,' she said.

'Thank you.'

'Do you want me to pull the curtains?' she offered. 'Perhaps you could have a little rest? You've been up all night, I hear.'

It was noisy on the ward, but somehow the curtains did block out the world a bit. Sorcha could hear the noise of the department, but for the first time since the gurney had slammed into her she was alone with her thoughts, and grateful that Richard had given her the space to be.

Monica came in and woke her a few hours later, still with Luke.

'Well, the ultrasound was normal,' she said. 'The placenta is nice and high, and the little one is unperturbed. You're twelve weeks pregnant, Sorcha. I know it was unplanned, but you're almost into your second trimester, so if you're considering not going ahead with the pregnancy...'

'I'm not having a termination.'

'Then congratulations,' Monica said. 'Your baby has a due date of June the tenth.'

Then Monica took a thorough history. There were a lot of questions, especially as she explained things to Luke along the way. They discussed everything from her uterus to her mental health and her accommodation.

'I think I'm staying at Richard's.'

'Okay,' Monica said. 'I'll sign you off work for two weeks and see you in clinic before you return.'

'I don't need that much time off—' Sorcha started, but then she sank back into the pillows. Maybe it would be better to have that time to sort things out with Richard. And even though she'd insisted she was fine, the events of today had upset her.

'These things can take a few days to catch up with you,' Monica said. 'You've had a proper fright. Still, I'm very happy with how things are—though you should bear in mind that you're going to be very tender from the bruising, so I want you to really try and rest over the next few days.' She checked her notes. 'I think that covers anything. Do you have any questions for me?'

Sorcha did. Because there was one question that hadn't been asked or answered.

When could she resume sex?

It was an odd question, because she hadn't had

sex in ages, and she was only staying at Richard's so they could sort out their cover story, but…

He was still the most attractive man she'd ever met…still the only person who could look right into her eyes and truly see her.

But Monica seemed to think the consultation was over.

Just as Monica walked off, Sorcha met the paramedic's eyes.

'Monica?' Luke said, and Monica turned. 'Sorry…' He was going through his notes. 'I must have missed it…when can the patient resume intercourse?'

'Oh!' Monica came back over. 'Sorcha, I'm sorry—I thought I'd said that. Sex is fine. As long as you're comfortable, of course.'

'Thanks,' Sorcha said, and the paramedic gave her a smile. 'Thanks,' she said a second time.

Not that she had any intention of finding out.

It was just good to know!

CHAPTER NINE

SORCHA CALLED RICHARD a short while after they'd gone.

'Monica said that the scan was perfect and she's happy. I can go home.'

'That's good. Have you thought about what I said?'

'Yes,' Sorcha said.

She'd thought about it a lot.

'I know it's a dreadful inconvenience…'

'I invited you,' Richard pointed out.

'If I could stay at yours that would be great.'

'Let's just take care of you for now.'

On leaving the hospital, Sorcha immediately regretted her decision to stay at Richard's. As the taxi drove them towards Canary Wharf she desperately wanted to change her mind and go to her crummy flat, or ask that he drive her the six hour journey to Scotland, but soon they were in an elevator.

'I'm on the nineteenth floor,' Richard said, as

the lift made pinging noises all the way up, then informed the occupants in an American accent that they'd reached floor nineteen.

'That voice drives me crazy,' Richard said as they stepped out into a hall with subdued lighting. 'I'm in apartment six.' He took out some keys. 'I just got this cut for you; I'd better make sure that it works.'

It did, and just as she was thinking once again that it had been a huge mistake to agree to staying here, the door opened to a view of London that had her breath catching in her throat.

'Welcome,' he said.

And he did just that. He made her feel incredibly welcome.

The view was incredible, but for now she just took in the soft, long leather couch and easy chair, and the low coffee table. It was a large lounge area, yet the artwork and the rug made it feel warm and inviting.

'I can smell polish,' Sorcha said, sniffing the lemony smell of beeswax in the air. 'Did you get a cleaner in?'

'I tried to.' He gave a wry laugh. 'She was booked out today so I had to do what I could.'

'It looks gorgeous.' She smiled.

'You won't be needing to see that for now,' Richard said, pointing towards a very plush-looking kitchen with black work surfaces. And then he gestured to a large study. 'Or that.'

He led her down a long hall.

'That's my room at the end...'

He hadn't closed the door and she could see a large unmade bed.

His bed.

She averted her eyes and he pushed open a second door. 'It's been a bit of a store room until today...'

'It's lovely.'

It really was. She even had her own bathroom which, after weeks of sharing the facilities at her flat, felt like the height of luxury.

'I've put a couple of my T-shirts and things in a drawer. I can go and collect some of your own clothes tomorrow, if you like.'

'I can do that.'

'No, you can't,' he said. 'You're here to get better. Just make a list. Or you can just make do for a few days. Now, what would you like for dinner?'

'I don't mind...whatever you're having.'

He took out his phone. 'I'm not offering to cook.'

'Pasta,' Sorcha said. 'But not loads.'

'Easy.'

He made what might have been awkward and difficult so easy.

'Right,' he said, once he'd ordered dinner. 'We're not talking about anything tonight.'

'You say that now…'

'I mean it,' he said. 'Under normal circumstances you'd have found out you were pregnant first, and then…' He shrugged. 'I don't know. However, you'd have had some time to come to grips with it.'

She nodded.

'So, let's keep to that. Unless you want to talk now?'

'Not yet.'

He'd made her feel so welcome, and now he was making what might have been a very difficult night so much easier.

Soon she was sitting on the sofa as Richard served up two bowls of creamy pasta carbonara, and she knew she wasn't waiting for him to pounce on her with questions.

They watched a spy show…a favourite of his.

'They all look normal,' Sorcha said.

'That's the point.'

It was a very sexy spy show, as it turned out, and watching that was possibly the only awkward moment between them.

'Sorry about that,' he said, taking her plate and rolling his eyes at the very sexy scene that they'd just had to sit through. 'Have you had enough to eat?'

'Plenty.'

'How's your stomach?'

'It's okay. I think I'll go to bed, though. I've hardly slept all day.'

'Of course.'

'I might have a shower first?'

'You don't have to ask permission.' He smiled. 'I got some shampoo and stuff for you.'

He had.

Shampoo for curly hair, and conditioner too!

It was nice to have a shower, but then she caught sight of her reflection as she stepped out and the vivid purple bruise high on her stomach made her breath catch. She thought of the little life within her and suddenly panicked, thinking how different things might have been.

'Don't go there,' she told herself aloud, drying off and then pulling on one of the T-shirts Richard had left for her.

She was so tired that she was certain she'd be asleep the moment she lay down, but instead she lay awake in the dark, with her mind racing back not just over the day's events, but over recent weeks.

How could she not have known she was pregnant?

She'd felt sick, and been dizzy a couple of times, but she'd been upset since that morning at the hotel.

Then she thought about what Monica had said—about it being close to decision time if she didn't want to go ahead with the pregnancy.

Would Richard want to discuss that?

She needed some water, and wished she'd thought to bring a glass to bed. She wondered about drinking from the tap in her bathroom, but that would be stupid when the kitchen was just down the hall.

'Hey…' Richard was standing at the living room window, looking out at the night, as she came out of her room.

'I was just getting a drink.'

'I meant to leave a jug of water and a glass in there…' He turned and smiled. 'My turn-down service isn't up to par.'

She filled a glass and took a long drink, then filled it again and walked over and looked out onto a night that had turned golden.

'Wow, look at all the lights.'

'I know,' he agreed. 'That's what sold it to me. I wasn't so sure—it used to all be offices around here. But the real estate agent was astute enough to bring me back at night.'

'It's so bright.' Sorcha gazed out and tried to get her bearings, looking at the black snake of river. 'Where's the hospital?'

'That way,' Richard said. 'And the palace is that way…'

She could see trains sliding into their stations like toys, and the whole of London was spread out before them.

'My flat in Scotland backs onto a huge park,' Sorcha said. 'The Glen—well, that's what the locals call it. There's just the tops of the trees and the sky...'

'Nice?'

'I could look at it for hours,' she admitted. 'I often do.'

'You miss it?'

'Yes.'

It wasn't homesickness that was troubling her now, though, and as she stared out at the endless buildings she wished she was good at broaching difficult topics.

She wasn't, though, so instead she blurted out what had been keeping her awake. 'You told me that you don't want children.'

He was silent for a moment before responding. 'Jess and I didn't...' He paused. 'Jess couldn't have children.'

'Oh.'

'She had a lot of gynae issues in her twenties.'

'I shouldn't have said anything.'

'Of course you should have. Look, it didn't seem fair to serve up her medical history whenever people asked, so we just said that it wasn't for us.'

'Might it have been? If she could have…?' Sorcha's voice trailed off. She knew her question was perhaps unfair. 'I'll say goodnight.'

'Night, Sorcha.'

Richard had been unsure how to answer that question and was grateful for the reprieve.

He lay on the sofa, looking out at the night, pondering Sorcha's question. Not so much whether he and Jess would have had a baby if they could have had one, but how he felt now that Sorcha was pregnant.

Having his baby.

For so long babies and children had been removed from the equation, and then a few short hours ago all that had changed.

He was going to be a father.

A parent.

How did it feel?

He didn't yet know.

The only thing he could say was that it didn't feel wrong.

Just very, very new…

Her first week at Richard's passed in a bit of a blur.

True to his word he didn't push for conversation about the pregnancy, but he brought her a mug of tea in the morning and they'd chat…

About how she'd slept.

How she felt.

'Better,' she said today, but then spoiled it by wincing as she sat up.

'Can I see?'

She nodded and lay back and lifted her T-shirt—or rather his T-shirt. It wasn't the first time he'd checked on her injury.

'Today's the worst day,' she said, and pulled the T-shirt down.

'Is it really sore?'

'More that it feels tender.' She shrugged. 'I didn't think it was that bad at the time. I get now why I'm here.'

'And why is that?'

'I'm pregnant with your baby.'

'I'm glad one of us has the answer.' Richard certainly didn't sound glad. 'Sorcha, that's a bit of an insult. I was concerned about you even before I knew about the baby.'

'You feel responsible.'

'I *am* responsible,' he retorted.

She squeezed her lips tight. Clearly he didn't know what he'd said wrong.

'That's actually a good thing, Sorcha,' he went on.

'Is it?'

It was the worst thing, Sorcha thought as she lay on her side, trying not to cry.

He was stuck with her.

As she was sure her parents felt they had been.

'Sorcha...' He came back a little while later and sat on the edge of the bed. 'We'll talk when you're ready. But know this... You're not on your own. You don't have to do this on your own. I know I'm not exactly ideal relationship material, but I will do everything I can to be there for the baby.'

'I know.'

It should help—and in many ways it did.

He was a very decent man and she knew he would do the right thing.

It was another piece of him she wanted, though. But that part belonged to someone else.

The second week brought things into sharper focus.

He collected her things from her awful flat and his silence was palpable as he handed her the holdall she'd been carrying on the day they'd met.

'Thanks.'

She didn't want his verdict on her flatmates and so she went through the bag, delighted to see her computer and all her personal effects.

'Why did you pack my bikini?'

'There's a pool here.'

'This isn't for swimming,' she said.

'What's it for?'

'Holidays,' Sorcha said. 'Lying by the pool.'

He smiled then, that serious face slipping away, and he melted her with the curve of his mouth and the little crinkle at his eyes.

'You're quite complicated, Sorcha.'

'I'm really not.'

'Oh, but you are.' He looked at her. 'We still haven't really spoken...'

'I know,' she said. 'I'm just trying to get my head around things.'

'Are you...?' He paused. 'Are you upset or...?'

'No,' Sorcha said. 'I'm still a bit stunned.'

'Did you ever picture yourself having children?' He gave her an apologetic smile. 'You did once ask me the same question.'

'I did,' she agreed. 'I don't know—and that's the truth. I wanted to sort things out with Amanda. But I'm not good at getting close to anyone, really. I know we fell into bed, but that really was an exception for me.'

'And for me.'

'Come on,' she said. 'You're not looking for anything serious.'

'I wasn't looking, full stop,' Richard said. 'Sorcha, you seem to think I was out on the pull that night?'

'No.' She shook her head. 'But I get it...' She shrugged.

'What?'

'Well, you come to London for a break, and...'

'I come to London to work, and sometimes I catch up with friends.' He frowned. 'You're the only person I've slept with since Jess's accident.' He frowned and she thought perhaps she wore a disbelieving expression. 'Is that so hard to accept?' he asked.

'It's been three years.'

'Three hellish years.' He nodded.

She inhaled sharply 'I thought…'

'Don't think. Ask,' Richard said. 'And when you're ready to talk, we'll do so.'

They did talk—though not about the issue. They spoke about so much, and Richard found himself liking their mornings together. And he was aware of a slight twitch to his lips when she said goodnight and headed to bed.

He'd sworn never to get involved again.

Not just out of loyalty.

More self-preservation.

Yet there was another heartbeat in his home. Two, in fact. And despite it being winter, the world felt warmer. Sorcha returned to work but there was no mention of her returning to her dreadful flat share, and for that Richard was very grateful. Instead, they'd settled into a comfortable routine. Days quickly passed, with both of them working their shifts and spending time together when not at work.

There was colour back in his life…literally.

Sorcha pointed out every rainbow.

'A double one…' she'd say, and he'd come out of his study and take a look.

There were also pastel-coloured knickers and bras tumbling in his dryer.

He came home from a very brief trip to Wales and his heart felt like lead.

No, he did not want to fall in love again.

It bloody hurt.

'What on earth…?'

There was a real Christmas tree in his lounge room, dressed in silver tinsel and red baubles, and there were reindeer on his marble countertops and a gingerbread house.

'Happy Christmas!' Sorcha smiled. 'I couldn't help myself.'

In truth, she'd been antsy all day, knowing where he was.

'How was the visit?' she made herself ask.

'It was okay,' he said.

They cooked pasta together and ate it in the dark, aside from the blaze of London and the twinkling tree.

'Do you have plans for Christmas?' he asked suddenly.

'I'm on an early, and then I'm spending the evening at Amanda's. What about you?'

'I'll go to my sister's on Christmas Eve, and then on to Wales Christmas morning. Are you looking forward to it?'

'I don't know,' Sorcha admitted. 'I want it to be incredible and…' She gave a soft laugh. 'I want her to love me, I guess.'

He smiled at her honesty.

'And not just a little bit,' Sorcha said. 'I want her flat all decorated for me, with mince pies and chestnuts laid out. My parents do all that…'

'Are you maybe looking for love in all the wrong places?'

He made her smile as he addressed the permanent ache in her heart.

'Probably,' Sorcha said, and she looked over to Richard and realised he could be more than a little bit right.

She loved sitting here with him.

As much as she had loved sitting with him at Kings Cross and watching the world go by.

'Are *you* looking forward to Christmas?' she asked.

'I like catching up with my sister and seeing her kids.'

'What about when you're in Wales?'

'We have decorations and mince pies and all this forced joviality.' He thought for a moment. 'I wonder what we'll be doing next year?'

She knew he was trying to broach the subject—

to get even a glimpse of what was going on inside her head—but Sorcha said nothing.

'Do you want to go out?' Richard suggested.

'When?'

'Now,' Richard said. 'We can go and see the Christmas lights.'

'It's late,' Sorcha said.

'Next year might be full of teething and babysitters.'

'I would love to see the lights.'

They walked down Oxford Street and Sorcha thought it was wonderful to be in London again. Or was it simply wonderful that she was looking at the Christmas lights with him?

'We'll do the tour,' Richard said.

It was an open top bus tour of London at night, and they sat on the open-top deck. But even with his arm around her and the dreadful woolly hats they'd quickly purchased, it was only just above freezing.

'Look at that…' They saw the London Eye, all lit up in pink, and the Shard, and then they travelled on to Westminster.

They reached Buckingham Palace and she saw the balcony. 'Do you do this every year?'

'I don't do this sort of thing ever. I only like doing these things with you.'

'What things?'

'Silly things.'

They got back to his flat and ate the hot chestnuts they'd bought from a stand, and then on Sorcha's demand he got out photos of him as a baby.

'Gosh, you were born serious!' She laughed, because, honestly, he was almost scowling in all the pictures.

It felt a lot like a first date.

Or a second or third.

But with no kisses.

They were trying, both of them, to take things slowly.

CHAPTER TEN

Christmas Eve

RICHARD WOKE AND it actually felt like Christmas Eve.

He could hear carols playing and Sorcha singing, and something better-smelling than muffins was baking in the oven.

He peeked in and saw there were fat sausages wrapped in bacon roasting. Very possibly it was the perfect breakfast.

He knocked on her bedroom door.

'Wait!' Sorcha said, and he rolled his eyes as he heard her moving things around. 'Okay, now you can come in.'

She was sitting on the bed, wrapping a huge box of candles.

'Does that mean I have to get you a present?' he asked.

He saw the flash of disappointment on her face and smiled. He knew what he'd bought for her, and he was actually looking forward to being back here with her on Boxing Day.

'What time do you head off?' Sorcha asked.

'Late afternoon—traffic will be bad. Are you going to stay at Amanda's today?'

'No.' Sorcha shook her head. 'I'll go there from work tomorrow. I'm just going to drop the presents off now, and the piggies in blankets.'

'I can smell them. I was knocking to ask if there were any available for us.'

'They should be ready.'

It was a gorgeous Christmas Eve breakfast, but all too soon it was time for Sorcha to go. And for Richard it felt as if Christmas was over already.

'I'll see you on Boxing Day,' he said.

'You shall.' Sorcha smiled. 'And then we've got a whole week off.'

'I hope it goes well with Amanda.'

'So do I.' She smiled. 'Happy Christmas.'

He wanted to kiss her—but then he always did.

Actually, he would like to cancel Christmas—at least the one that was planned—and haul Sorcha to bed and turn off his phone.

Instead, he loaded the car with presents for Jess and her family, as well as for his sister and the little ones.

The motorway was surprisingly clear for Christmas Eve, but it didn't offer him relief. He felt as if he was hurtling in the wrong direction.

'Richard!'

Gemma was delighted to see him, and it was great to see the kids, but his smile slipped as his sister put her overexcited children to bed and he stared out of the black kitchen window.

'I know.' His sister's hand came on his shoulder. 'It's a difficult time.'

She was offering him support, only it felt undeserved. Her assumption that he was pensive tonight because of Jess was wrong, and he didn't want to milk things. Ever.

'It's not Jess,' Richard said. 'I've met someone.'

'Richard?' He could hear the shock in Gemma's voice. 'I had no idea you were even back out there.'

'Nor did I,' he admitted. 'Her name's Sorcha.'

'And where is she now?'

'Either about to have the best Christmas or the worst,' Richard said. 'And I feel I should be there with her.'

Sorcha was having the worst Christmas.

A text to Amanda had bounced back, and she was having a sense of déjà-vu as she saw the full mailbox at Amanda's flat.

She knocked, and knocked again, and then a man came out with a little dog.

'Amanda's not here.'

'I can see.' Sorcha smiled. 'I just wanted to drop these off. Do you know when she'll be back?'

'She moved out at the weekend.'

Sorcha fired off another text and almost folded in relief as Amanda swiftly responded.

At least until she read it.

Undeliverable.

She'd been blocked.

Again.

It wasn't like last time, Sorcha told herself as she clattered down the stairs. She was older, and she had gone into this with eyes wide open. She'd known there wouldn't be rainbows and unicorns...

But the pep talks didn't help.

And all she knew was that she wasn't wanted.

Again.

It felt as if her heart was a dartboard, with all the little stings of shame, but somehow she got through her shift. When she let herself into the flat, she didn't even turn the Christmas lights on.

She didn't understand... Why had Amanda got in touch just to do this again?

And what was she, Sorcha, doing here when she had a family in Scotland?

The only reason she was here now was Richard.

And the only reason she was here in Richard's home was the baby they'd made.

She wasn't going to tell him what had happened. Sorcha made her decision as she fell asleep and woke up feeling the same way.

The streets were empty—that was the only good thing about Christmas morning, Sorcha decided. But she smiled and wished everyone Happy Christmas, and pulled crackers with the night staff, and then she dealt with a croupy baby and saw him up to the children's ward.

It was a happy place to be on Christmas morning, and Sorcha smiled as she watched a huge rabbit giving out gifts.

'Isn't that the Easter Bunny?' David, the porter, frowned.

'Shush.' Sorcha smiled. 'He's wearing tinsel.'

It was when she got back to the unit that things fell apart.

'Phone for you, Sorcha,' called one of her colleagues.

'Sorcha speaking?'

'Happy Christmas.'

The voice was unexpected. She'd been expecting it to be the path lab, with some results she'd been chasing, but it was Richard.

'I tried your mobile.'

'It's in my locker.'

'I realised that. Is it busy there?'

'No,' Sorcha said. 'It's actually quiet. How's your day?'

'Quiet,' Richard said. 'How's Amanda?'

'I'm going there tonight.'

'I hope she appreciated the sausages yesterday.'

'Yes.' Sorcha pressed her thumb and forefinger into her eyes. 'She did...'

But she knew her voice was croaky and that he must have noticed.

'Sorcha?'

'She's...'

'What?'

'Please don't ask,' Sorcha said. 'I have to work.'

'Are you seeing Amanda tonight?'

'No,' Sorcha said. 'But I think I knew it was coming. I have to go...'

As terrible Christmases went, it was getting worse...

'It's croup city,' May said, and sure enough here were two more babies, barking like little seals.

'She's okay,' Sorcha said to one anxious mum. 'I know it sounds dreadful...'

'It sounded worse at home.'

'The damp air outside helps.'

The Easter Bunny was still masquerading as Santa Bunny when she took one of the baby seals up to the ward, and there was a puppet show too. She stayed to watch for a few moments and saw the staff making such an effort.

The consultants were wearing Santa hats, and there were smiles on some of the parents' faces as they sat by their very ill children's bedsides, and that made her own problems less.

The gratitude stayed with her. Sorcha even wore her flashing earrings on the way home and then let herself into the empty flat.

Only it wasn't so empty. It smelt spicy and delicious as she stepped in, and the lights on the tree were on.

'Hello?' she called, and was startled as Richard appeared.

'Happy Christmas,' he said.

'I thought you were being burgled.'

'Do you say hello to all home invaders?'

He smiled, and she both cried and laughed as she embraced him.

'What are you doing here?'

'It's where I want to be.'

'Is that a new jumper?' She ran a hand over grey cashmere. 'It's very nice…'

And then she realised she was stroking his chest. And it felt as if her hand had got stuck… as if the cashmere turned to Velcro. And she had to pull it back to remove it.

Oh, she shouldn't have touched him.

She truly hadn't meant to.

He politely pretended not to notice, and handed her a glass of alcohol-free mulled wine. 'It tastes dreadful—be warned!'

It did. But it was instantly her favourite drink.

'Come on,' he said, 'we are going to eat.'

Only he didn't pull out his phone, and there were no signs of recent deliveries as he led her to a beautifully dressed table, lit with red candles and decorated with holly, and laden with slices of turkey, ham, stuffing and all the trimmings.

'Gemma,' he said by way of explanation. 'I went begging.'

'Gemma's the pretty one?'

'Correct,' he said, and then confessed, 'I've told her.'

He pulled out a chair and she sat down.

'What did she say?' asked Sorcha.

'I've been fully lectured,' he said. 'I actually called you this morning because by the time I got to Wales I felt guilty for teasing you. Of course I'd got you a gift…'

She looked beneath the tree and there was a box. Medium-sized. And, no, she wasn't expecting a ring, but it looked very jewellery-ish, and there was another flat box by its side.

'Which one's mine?'

'Both,' Richard said. 'Sort of.'

'Can I open them now?'

'No.'

They ate, and it was a lot of food when she'd been grazing all day, but it was gorgeous to eat by candlelight.

But there was something she had to know.

'What about...?' She swallowed. 'What did you say to Jess's family?'

'I said I'd been called in to work.'

He knew it sounded a cop-out, and he wanted to explain that he knew decent people didn't ruin others' Christmas Day, but that would only hurt. So he didn't explain...

'What's this?' He looked at a large box that looked rather similar to the gift she'd wrapped for Amanda. 'Candles?'

'Open it.'

Sorcha was blushing, and wondering if she'd got his gift dreadfully wrong.

'A medical compendium?'

'With flash cards and all the bits...' she said. 'I don't know if it will help with your studies, or if I'm pushing...'

'You're not pushing,' he said. 'I'm going to go for it. The exam's in May, then the baby arrives in June.'

'I'm pleased.'

She smiled, and then it was her turn to open her gifts. She reached for the small one...the exciting-looking one.

'Open the other box first...'

It was all ribbons, and she tore at them, and

then at more paper, and then she opened the dark blue velvet box inside.

'Oh...'

It was a dress watch, silver, with gorgeous Roman numerals. When she put it on, he helped with the fiddly clip and it actually fitted.

'How did you manage to get my size?'

'Your hospital wristband,' he told her, revealing his devious ways.

'It's perfect.' She would remember them meeting every time she looked at her watch. 'When every second counts you tend to notice them.'

'Yes.'

He made every second count.

She opened the flat box, and found it was a tiny silver frame in the shape of a bell.

'A photo frame for the Christmas tree,' Richard said. 'I thought we could get a picture of us for the baby.'

She looked up.

'Whatever happens between us, our baby will know we mattered a lot to each other.'

'We did.'

She teared up, and then quickly went to put some lip balm on and let down her hair. She moved to take the flashing earrings out.

'Keep them in,' he said, and they went to sit on the couch and took a few photos, capturing their first Christmas.

She lay there scrolling through them.

'That one,' Richard said.

Only Sorcha didn't answer. Because she'd felt something like a little tickle, only stronger.

'It moved.'

'Sorcha—'

'It did.'

'You're only sixteen weeks…'

'Almost seventeen.'

He slipped up her top and looked at her stomach. It wasn't flat, even when she was lying down.

'I know I felt it,' Sorcha said. 'Like a little bird.'

'I can't feel anything,' he admitted. He knew the baby was too small to be felt just yet, but soon…

And then he saw the flash of red hair above her knickers.

And she was looking right at him as his fingers made light circles on her stomach.

And she was willing his hand to move down, just staring at his mouth and watching his lips press together.

And she didn't know that passion could be so instant.

'We agreed,' he said, pulling down her top. 'I gave you my word.'

'Even soldiers get an amnesty at Christmas.'

'We're not at war.'

'Exactly,' Sorcha said. And when he lowered his head and kissed her she felt every fear and every last bit of upset dissolve into nothing. His kiss was so slow and deep it chased everything other than this moment away.

'This isn't sensible,' he warned.

'I don't care.'

It felt right. It felt better than right.

He stripped off his cashmere and her Velcro hands were back, stroking his skin and the fan of hair on his chest. And then she was kissing his neck and his shoulders as he knelt on the floor and she sat up on the couch.

Between deep kisses they slipped out of their clothes, and he traced her newly pink areolae.

He gave her a sensual lover's kiss that made her sigh as his tongue slid in...a kiss that was thorough and faint-making. Their lower bodies were pressing together, his hands digging into her bottom... She could honestly have come just from this kiss.

'Don't stop...' she protested as he pulled back.

And then she realised she was yet to learn there was no stopping this. He pulled her towards the edge of the sofa and exposed her sex and all the gorgeous changes there. She was hot and swollen, and as she exposed him in return, holding him again, her head on his chest, her legs apart, she just wanted to touch the dark crinkly hair for a moment, and see the beauty of him.

Then he took over, moving her right to the edge of the couch, and slid in.

She knew the feel of her, oiled and gripping, must be wonderful for him, because he groaned, and she hovered on the edge of bliss.

They both watched themselves, and it was the most erotic thing she'd ever seen. And then her eyes closed and she put her hands behind her, leaning back, feeling one of his hands pressing into her, the other exploring her breasts. Her thighs were trembling, her calves were wrapped around him, and she felt the warm spread of him, heard the harsh breaths from him.

She buried her face in his neck, almost scared to allow her release. She dared not give in. She wanted to plead and beg him for for ever. There was a desperation rising in her and she knew that she might tell this zipped-up man who had only ever loved one woman that she was completely and utterly crazy about him.

Instead, she gave in to her climax and felt him unleash. And those last powerful thrusts as she came down from her own orgasm almost shot her up there again.

'It's going to be okay,' he told her as he lowered her down. 'Come with me.'

He led her to his bed and they lay there together. He wanted to tell her that there would be no more spare room.

Ever.

But it was too soon for that, surely?

Richard lay there, staring at the ceiling, and knew that if he'd found out three years ago he was to be father to the child of a woman he'd slept with once—or rather, twice now—he'd have laughed at the ridiculousness of the situation.

Now, he lay there and felt the swell of her stomach, inhaled the scent of her hair, and he felt as he had that morning back at the hotel.

It was a feeling he examined as he quietly lay there.

Happiness?

Oh, it wasn't smiling and whistling... It was something more. It was peaceful and yet thrilling. It was a new state of normal that he'd never thought he'd feel.

CHAPTER ELEVEN

AMNESTY WAS EXTENDED to New Year's Eve.

They saved all the questions for later and simply enjoyed each other as they got to know each other.

'We should go out,' Sorcha said. 'Celebrate. We might not be able to next year.'

'True,' Richard said.

'Mexican?'

Sorcha was wearing a clinging mint-green woollen dress and loads of coral lipstick and he thought he'd never seen her go all out like that before.

And he would like to stay in.

'Spanish-Mexican?' Richard said. 'It's a restaurant at the hotel we stayed at for the conference. I wanted to try it…'

'Okay.'

'And there are views…'

'There are views here,' Sorcha pointed out, having possibly read his mind.

But it was brilliant to go out.

To be just another couple and unburdened.

'Happy New Year,' Richard said at midnight.

'Happy New Year.'

They kissed, and then they danced on a tiny dance floor, so small and crowded that there was no other way to dance than to get really close.

So close...

He breathed in her hair, that coconut scent, and he tried not to compare. But therein was the issue.

There was no comparison.

He'd been in love once, and very deeply. It had been a gorgeous, steady, slow burn.

This love—and he was almost sure that was what it was—was like a white-hot flame that danced and flickered and shot life back into his dead heart.

But he would never declare it until he was certain...

The evening before Sorcha's twenty-one-week scan they lay in bed, the world blocked out with his industrial blackout blinds, talking about the next day.

'Do you want to find out what we're having?' she asked.

'I don't mind,' he admitted.

'Do you care what we have?'

'I care,' Richard said. 'Though not about what

we have.' He asked her a question. 'When are you going to tell your parents?'

'In a couple of weeks.'

'Good.'

'When are you going to tell yours?'

'I don't know.'

'What did Gemma say?'

He didn't answer. It wasn't just Sorcha being evasive. Gemma had warned him it was all too much too soon. And not to make promises he couldn't keep and rush into commitment. It wasn't just Gemma who'd voiced her doubts—word had spread through the hospital and a few friends had attempted gentle, cautious words...

He didn't want to tell Sorcha all that.

'She said not to rush you,' he told her.

'You haven't rushed me,' Sorcha said, and then took a deep breath. 'But I don't want to be second best.'

She had to ask. Had to know.

'Would we be lying here now if I wasn't pregnant?'

'Would we be lying her now if the trains hadn't been cancelled?' Richard countered.

'It's not the same,' Sorcha said. 'I don't want you to feel stuck with me.'

'What if I want to be stuck with you?'

'Would you come to Scotland?'

He didn't answer.

'The thing is, I don't know if I want to live here,' she admitted as they lay in the dark. 'I have family and friends back home.'

She closed her eyes. It wasn't just that. It was the thought of only having part of him. And she knew there were difficult times ahead. He'd been to Wales again today. Jess was having increasing seizures and that feeling in the pit of her stomach was back.

She was scared that one day he'd look over at her and realise it wasn't the right woman in his bed. Or, worse, he'd think it but be too damn honourable to say it.

But she'd know.

'*Would* you move to Scotland?' she asked.

'Sorcha, it's seven hours on a train from Edinburgh to Wales. We're talking fourteen hours travel in a day...'

'But if I asked?'

'It would mean a lot more of my time spent on trains...' He stroked her arm. 'I'd hoped you wouldn't ask just yet.'

'I see.' She took a breath. 'I know that you and Jess successfully lived in separate places...'

'It's not the same.'

'Is it because of the baby?'

'No.' He shook his head.

'Jess, then.' She breathed out. 'So I'd have to sort my family, my home, my childcare around—'

'Sorcha.' He stopped her from being mean. 'You know those guys who say they'll move heaven and earth for a woman?'

'Yes...'

'They're lying. Because no one can move heaven and earth. But I will do what I can to be there for you if you choose to live in Scotland.'

She wanted the heaven and earth guy, though. Not the logical, honest one.

Richard did not know the right answer. He felt this terrible grip in his chest when he thought of dividing himself between three countries and not being able to get to either of them enough.

No, it wasn't about the baby.

And yet...

Another person to worry about, to love...

'I'm sorry,' she said.

'Don't be. We need to talk.'

'I love my flat in Scotland,' she said. 'And not just the building. I came to London to sort things with Amanda and she's taken off. I've only got you here.'

'Okay...'

'I don't see the point of being in a flat a few miles from here...'

'What about moving in with me?' He turned to her and even in the dark saw her eyes widen.

'We haven't known each other for long enough.' She shook her head. 'That doesn't sound very...'

'What?'

They were both trying to be honest, lying there in bed and trying to sort things out, but they just chased in circles.

Sorcha was trying to hold on to her heart.

Richard was unsure if he was in a place to receive it, let alone if he even had a heart he dared give.

'We could just stay in bed for the next few months,' she said. 'Eat chocolate and make love.'

'That sounds incredible,' Richard said, but then he flicked open the blackout blinds. 'But I have to go to work so I can pay for my rail card...'

She laughed.

And somehow he liked it that he made her laugh even on those difficult days, and in those difficult conversations, and he kissed her goodbye before heading in for his night shift.

'Haemorrhoids,' May told him. 'Cubicle seven.'

'Thank you.'

'Richard,' she said, in that low tone that meant she was about to get personal. 'Can I ask you something?'

He liked May, he really did, but if one more

person told him he was moving too fast and that he was heading for a crash, or not to make promises he couldn't keep...

He would never make a promise he couldn't keep.

'Of course,' he said to May.

'I've got blood in my urine.'

He turned. 'How much blood?'

'A lot. I just went to the toilet...' She was teary and flustered. 'A *lot*!'

'Come on,' he said, 'we'll go to Mr Field's office.'

'You're sure?'

'So long as you're not going to faint,' he said. 'You haven't been eating beetroot, have you?' he teased as they walked around to the offices.

'Jesus!' she said, and started wailing as Richard frowned. 'Why didn't I think of that...?' She started to laugh. 'I had it for lunch—with walnuts and feta.'

She started to laugh, and so did he, and the oddest part for him—the truly new part—was that he couldn't wait to get home and tell Sorcha the story.

It was silly, and funny, and as they headed back all he wanted was to call her...to wake her up just to tell her he missed her tonight.

He got back to work and was mid examination when he heard a commotion outside.

There was the shout of a parent's pure fear that he'd know anywhere, but then he was relieved to hear the sound of a child crying. Vanessa and May were with them, though he kept his ears pricked and heard the parents explaining that their baby had vomited.

'Fainted?' a woman said in broken English.

'She's okay,' he heard Vanessa reassure them, but he concluded his examination and, instead of taking bloods, told the patient he'd be back shortly.

The urgent shout that had alerted him was hard to shake off. 'What have you got?' he asked Vanessa, who was now at the nurses' station.

'Gastro,' she said. 'She's fine. She's had a few bowel actions overnight, and a vomit this morning. She's a little bit dehydrated. I'm going to start an IV... I'm just waiting for the numbing gel to take effect.'

'Perhaps bring her over to Resus?' May suggested. 'Mum's ever so upset.'

'I don't think all that equipment will help her to calm down,' Vanessa countered.

'But from the history the little one might have had a seizure.'

'Fine,' Vanessa said, but with a slight edge that told May she thought she was overreacting.

As May went to move the family, Richard knew he should butt out, but he couldn't.

'If May's worried...' he said. 'If any of the nursing staff are worried...' He breathed in, seeing Vanessa's features pinch, but he didn't get to finish the conversation because it was then that panic returned to the department.

The mother let out another dreadful wail and Vanessa jumped down from her stool, dashing out. Richard followed her, truly expecting to see the baby seizing or collapsed, but instead she was completely fine, patting her distraught mother's cheeks.

'It's okay,' May attempted to soothe the distressed mother. 'We just want to keep a closer eye on little Dina...'

Then the lady's knees buckled. But a very deft May must have seen it coming, because she dealt with it rapidly, as did the baby's father, guiding the mother to a seat.

In the midst of the confusion Richard was left holding the baby.

'Are you going to vomit on me?' he asked little Dina as May helped the mother, who was wearing just a nightdress beneath her coat.

He looked to the father, who was trying to calm his wife down even though he had tears streaming down his own cheeks.

'Sir?' Richard said, and the man looked up. 'Shall we go and talk somewhere else?' When he nodded, Richard smiled at the little girl, who was now openly staring at him. 'I'm going to talk to your daddy...'

'I'll take her.' May held out her arms and the very cute little girl went easily into them. 'Oh, Richard—she's waving to you!'

'Pardon?'

'She's waving to you.'

He didn't really do the baby thing, but she was exceptionally cute... Or was it that he'd be a father himself soon? Whatever the reason, he gave Dina a wave back, then led the father to one of the family rooms.

Richard introduced himself and asked the man's name.

'Tony,' he said, and cleared his throat.

'You're Dina's father?' he checked—because if the years had taught him anything, it was never to assume. 'You're Dina's parents?'

'Yes,' he said. 'Shula is my wife... Dina's mother.'

'What's been going on, Tony?'

'She went all floppy...'

'Did you see that happen?'

'No, my wife screamed and I ran and got the car...' He was calming down now, and took two rapid intakes of breath, then slowly exhaled. 'We lost our son...'

'How old was he?'

'Six months.'

'When did that happen?'

'He'd be ten now.' Tony gave a helpless, defeated shrug. 'We brought him here, to this hospital...that same room.'

'I'm so sorry,' Richard said. 'I know this is difficult, but I do have to ask you some questions.'

Tony nodded.

'What was the cause of death?'

'Sudden infant death...' he said. 'They couldn't tell us why. I said to the doctor just now, when she asked, that Dina was an only child. I didn't want to upset my wife. You can see how she gets.'

'Yes...' Richard paused. 'We do need to know, though.'

'I was going to tell the doctor away from my Shula.' He looked at Richard. 'Nothing can happen to Dina. We weren't ever going to have another baby; we both swore we could never go through it again.'

Richard nodded.

'When she screamed, I thought it had happened again.'

'Of course.'

'Does Dina have to be in that room?'

'She does.' Richard knew he sounded like a cold bastard, but he wasn't going to stop monitoring the baby just to appease the parents. 'We need to keep a close eye on her. And that means putting her on a cardiac monitor. If you stay calm it will help.'

'Yes.'

He went with Tony back into Resus and the mother gave him a pale smile. Dina was bouncing around on her lap.

'She's looking bright,' he said, watching the little girl who was smiling and utterly without a care. 'We're just going to pop her onto a monitor.'

'No...'

'It's nothing to be scared of.'

Richard took a couple of sticky dots from the trolley and handed one to Dina, who seemed delighted by it, and May soon had them on her chest and her pyjama top back down. He looked at the screen, pleased to see normal rhythm, but still concerned.

He brought Vanessa up to speed on the situation.

'They told me she was an only child.'

'I know they did,' Richard agreed. 'Let's get the brother's notes and see where we're at.'

'Do you think the episodes are related?'

'I sincerely hope not,' Richard said, 'but it's a possibility. I'm worried her electrolytes are out, and maybe that's caused an arrythmia.'

As Vanessa went to see another patient he looked over to the little family. Dina looked up and caught his eye and waved.

He duly waved back.

'Look at you,' May teased, 'waving to babies. I've got the brother's notes for you.'

She was busy trying to get some blood labs back, and she tapped away on the computer as he read through the brother's history.

'I remember him,' May said. 'It was awful.'

'Doctor!' Tony shouted. 'She's vomiting.'

'It's okay,' Richard said, making his way over.

May was straight on it, recording a heart trace and he watched the mother talking to her baby, trying to stay calm as she retched.

'She's okay,' he said again, even when Dina went pale and limp.

He took the baby and placed her on the bed.

'Do you want me to fast-page Paeds?' May asked, but he shook his head. Dina was opening her eyes.

'Hello,' he said to the little girl, who'd now started crying. 'You don't like vomiting, do you?'

It looked like a vasovagal; Dina had been holding her breath as she retched. But with the family history he would have to give his findings to the paediatricians.

He looked over to May. 'Call George for me and ask if he can come down…' George was the paediatric consultant on call tonight, and Richard knew that, if he was able to, he would come straight down.

'You can hold her,' he said to Shula, and she scooped the little girl into her arms.

Richard wrote his notes up by the bed, ordered some bloods and a chest X-ray, and then stood when George arrived.

'Dina's been scaring her parents,' Richard said.

'So I've heard.' George smiled at them and they went through the events of the night and looked at the heart tracing taken during the event.

'May told you about their son?' Richard checked.

'She did.' George nodded. 'Ashrim.'

Richard left the little family in George's very capable hands, and was just heading off to get changed when Mr Field stopped him.

'Richard,' he said, 'have you a moment?'

'Of course.'

It was unexpected—but then life so often was.

Mr Field asked him if he'd registered for the FRCEM exam, and Richard told him he had. 'It's in May.'

'Have you thought about a permanent role here?' Mr Field asked. 'I'm not retiring—it's Mr Owen who is.'

'Oh...'

'Don't listen to rumours.'

'I know.'

'So, is it something that might be on your radar?'

'Absolutely,' Richard said, responding with

confidence even if he wasn't sure it was feasible. 'However, I should—'

'Just give it some thought,' Mr Field interrupted. 'It's something to think about.'

'Yes.'

Richard was flattered—especially after the rollercoaster of recent years—and a permanent role at The Primary was more than he'd dared consider.

It wasn't just about him, though.

How could he ask Sorcha to stay here in London when it wasn't where she wanted to be?

He felt the shudder of his heart trying to grind back into life, and didn't see how he could make things work.

He couldn't even ask her to be his wife.

Richard stopped by the ambulance bay and stood there, going through all the reasons it was impossible.

He'd been told by everyone and anyone not to rush things.

Don't make promises you can't keep.

Told that he was still grieving…

'Doctor…?'

He looked over and there was Tony.

'How's Dina?'

'They're going to take her up to the children's ward soon.' He gave him a tired smile. 'Doctor George is quite sure she is holding her breath—

cheeky girl.' He smiled again. 'He wants to run some tests, though, and be very sure. I think Shula feels better.'

'What about you?'

'I don't know yet.' Tony sighed. 'Do you have children?'

'No,' he said, and then he did something he usually didn't. 'Not yet, but we're expecting a baby in June.'

It felt odd to say 'we', but he didn't know how else to say that he was soon to be a father.

'Congratulations.'

'Thank you.'

Richard smiled. Tony was the first person to say it.

Everyone else had been shocked, or worried, or warning him to be careful. It was nice to simply be congratulated.

'Do you know what you're having?' Tony asked.

'No, we've got an ultrasound later today.'

And he wasn't one for opening up—not at all—but he admired this man who stood next to him, who'd been brave enough to risk having a child again—and, hell, he could use some help.

'Can I ask you a question?' Richard said. 'It's personal…you don't have to answer.'

'Sure.'

'You said you didn't want another baby?'

'We didn't.' Tony shook his head. 'Neither of us wanted that pain again. We didn't think we could survive it.'

Richard nodded, wondering if Dina had been an accident.

'Ashrim brought us love and hope and so much laughter...' Tony paused. 'And then suddenly, it was gone.' He paused again, then said, 'We still had love and hope and laughter, but it was very...' His hand moved as he tried to summon the words. 'Not as strong.'

Richard smiled. 'Yes.' He understood that, because after Jess's accident life had carried on, and he had been happy at times, still lived, but it had all felt...

'Diluted?' Tony said. 'My English is not so good.'

'Your English is incredible.'

Diluted was the word that had eluded Richard for three years, but it was the perfect one now. When grief was strong, joy was dimmed, diluted...

But no longer.

Over the last few years he'd looked forward to the escape of work. But now, while still enjoying work, he was looking forward to going home. To finding a treat Sorcha might have left, or to a mug of tea being placed in front of him, or to sitting with her at night, just talking.

There were undeniable problems ahead, though—and he couldn't see a solution.

'Yet you decided to try again?' he said to Tony.

'Not straight away. It was not an easy decision. All our family pressured us… "Have another baby," they said. "Try again." But we both…'

He paused, and Richard found his ears were straining, aching to hear how these people who had lost so much had known it was time to try again.

'We didn't think we could love another baby as much as our first…' He rolled his eyes. 'But you have met our beautiful daughter.'

'Indeed,' Richard said. 'She's gorgeous.'

'I knew,' he said. 'And Shula knew too.'

Richard frowned, the answer still eluding him. 'Knew what?'

'I don't know how to explain it…' Tony apologised. 'We just knew.'

CHAPTER TWELVE

AND RICHARD KNEW.

His life had been diluted.

And then triple-strength concentrated red cordial had come along—or rather Sorcha had—and turned the word as he knew it on its head.

He didn't need all the doubters, or to be warned to proceed with caution. Life was a chance to be taken...

The shops were open by the time he got out of work, and he went for coffee and made a few calls. He was just stepping onto the escalator for the Tube and heading for home when Trefor called.

'Hey...' Richard said. He was halfway down the escalator, his phone starting to cut out. 'I'm coming this weekend—'

'Come now!' Trefor yelled, and his tone was filled with the same shrill panic that had shot his nerves to alert this morning, when Dina had come in. 'Now!'

Richard had known for three years that this

day would come, and had prepared for it as best he could. But now, when he heard Jess's latest dire observations, he still felt completely unprepared...

He had run for many trains—knew the schedule almost off by heart. And he spilled onto the concourse, bought his ticket, ran for the barrier and boarded the train for Cardiff.

'Richard...'

It was Jess's doctor on the phone now, and he was calm and brilliant, and by Jess's bedside, talking him through another prolonged seizure.

'We're giving her another five of Midazolam...'

The countryside was zipping by and soon he spoke with Trefor again.

'She's not doing well, Richard. What time will—?'

Then his phone cut out.

Richard stared at the black screen and tried to turn it back on. But then realised it had run out of charge.

Not now.

He asked a lady if he could borrow her charger, but she gave him such a startled look he moved on to the next person.

And he knew he must look like a mad man, because everyone looked away or avoided him.

'Sorry...'

Richard hadn't forgotten the ultrasound, or that he was meant to be meeting Sorcha.

But there were times when there was nothing you could do, and there was no right answer, nothing that could make things right...

This was his life. And it wasn't as if he hadn't told Sorcha how grave things were and how quickly they might change.

Yes, he would miss the ultrasound. He just hoped that Sorcha would understand.

Sorcha didn't understand.

Richard hadn't come home—but then again, his shifts sometimes went way over.

She was early, she reasoned, lining up at the Radiology desk.

'Sorcha Bell,' she told the receptionist.

'Take a seat.'

There were couples sitting together, and women sitting alone. Of course she didn't need him to be there.

She just wanted him to be.

More, she'd thought Richard wanted to be here for this, too.

She fired him a text—a happy, light-hearted one to say that she'd arrived—and then she waited...

Nothing came back.

Her appointment time came and went.

She stared at her phone, willing him to reply to her texts, or for him to call, but there was nothing.

He's an emergency doctor, she told herself. *Delays are to be expected.*

Something must have come up.

It didn't help to think it might be Jess.

The love of his life.

He and Jess had been together for fifteen years before the accident.

Sorcha sat there in the waiting room doing the maths.

For her and Richard to get there he'd have to be fifty and she'd be in her forties, and she felt silly for thinking she could ever come close to what he and Jess had had.

'Sorcha Bell?'

She looked up as her name was called and nodded, then made her way to the cubicle.

'Is it just you?' the radiographer asked, and Sorcha nodded again.

'Yes.'

She was on her own.

And it was time to get used to it.

Her dress was the worst possible choice to wear for having an ultrasound, and she rolled it up and lay there, feeling like a sausage roll that had burst open.

But then an image came on the screen.

'Is that…?'

Of course it was her baby—but it was incredible, seeing the little face and lips, just so detailed, legs that kicked and tiny slender feet.

Richard should be here!

What was the point of her being in London if he couldn't be here for moments such as this?

'Do you want to know what you're having?'

'No.' Sorcha shook her head. 'We wanted it to be a surprise.'

'Look away, then, because the baby's moving.'

She turned her head away and stared at the wall, but suddenly she was tired of uncertainty.

'Actually...' She changed her mind. 'I would like to know.'

It was a wonderful moment, and she cried out in surprise. She would have loved to reach into the screen to hold her little one. But that sweet moment was over too soon, and she was back on the busy London streets, and she had to double-check the map to make sure she was going in the right direction for Canary Wharf.

Suddenly she was tired of being a little bit lost in London.

Fed up with chasing people who didn't fully want her, or couldn't commit.

She took a breath. She knew Richard wouldn't appreciate being lumped into the same category as Amanda... Right now, though, he was. And she had to preserve her heart and be strong for her little one.

She put a hand over her not so small bump.

'We're going home.'

Jess was okay.

Not well, but not as bad as Richard had envisaged on the hellish journey there.

He knew the day was coming, though.

It might be tomorrow, it might be in ten years, but he would be there for her—as he'd promised.

'You gave us a fright,' Richard said gently, holding Jess's hand. 'But it's all okay now. Get some rest.'

He glanced up as Trefor came in and gave him a pale smile.

'How's she doing?' Trefor asked.

'She's resting.'

'Is your phone working now?'

'It is. They're charging it at the nurses' station.'

He'd seen the many missed calls and had fired Sorcha a text, explaining that Jess had been taken very ill...

But he knew something had to give.

'I'll have to head off soon,' he said.

'Already?'

'Yes.'

He could blame work again, but that had been a Christmas lie, and he loved Trefor and Bronwyn too much to have them inadvertently find out. They deserved far better. And even though he would do anything not to hurt them, life had already taken care of that.

'I'm just going to speak with your dad,' he said to Jess, and then kissed her hot forehead. 'I'll be back soon.'

He motioned to Trefor.

'What's this all about?' he asked as Richard headed to one of the small sitting rooms.

'Trefor...' Richard took a seat, but Trefor stood. 'I haven't told anyone apart from Gemma, but I don't want you to hear this from anyone else.'

'What's that, then?'

'I've met someone.'

Trefor shot him a look. 'I could have saved you a confession. We knew you were seeing someone at Christmas, when you legged it out of here before lunch.'

Richard let that one go. 'We're having a baby.'

His father-in-law's reaction was just as swift and below the belt as the last. 'Well, you didn't waste much time, did you?' Trefor sneered.

Richard let that one go too, and chose not to mention that it had been three years, because he knew his father-in-law well and could already see there were tears in his eyes.

'Oh, God...' Trefor suddenly sobbed. 'A baby...'

Trefor sat down then and wept, and Richard stayed with him. 'I know it's hard...'

'You don't know!' he said, then relented. 'Of course you do.' He was a mess. 'Will you still come and see our Jess?'

'Trefor...' Richard did not let that one go. 'Look at me.' He waited until Trefor did so. 'Do you need to ask?'

He'd known Trefor since he was eighteen and Trefor had known him.

'You know that I'll still be coming here, but I'm telling you now because I'll need to be there for Sorcha too.'

'You're right.' Trefor was blowing his nose and sniffing, calming down. But this man had almost lost his daughter today. 'Oh, Richard. You a father!'

'I'll be back here in a few days,' Richard said. 'But if you need a bit of a break from me, I'll understand. We need to honest.'

'Yes.' Trefor nodded. 'I appreciate that.'

Sorcha had got Richard's text, but it felt too late for all that. She ran up the escalator at the station and this time around there wasn't a single person blocking her way.

She got a ticket in moments and there were no cancellations...

Nothing to stop her from heading straight onto the train and home.

Except the baby was kicking—real kicks—as

if in protest, and it was those little kicks that had her slowing down and drawing in breath.

She didn't want to go, she wanted to stay, but more than that she wanted Richard's love.

Wanted to be the love of his life.

It was hard to accept he'd already had that when she was head over heels in love with him.

But maybe love really did make you brave, because now she did something she'd never thought she would.

Sorcha took out her phone, drew in a breath and called him.

'Hello?' he said.

'How's Jess?' she asked.

'She's stable now...just resting,' he said. 'Did you get my message?'

'About two hours after I had the ultrasound I got one that said your phone had died.'

'How did it go?'

'It went well,' she said, but didn't elaborate. 'Where are you now?'

'About half an hour from Paddington. Where are you?'

'I'm already at Kings Cross.'

'What time's your train?' he said with an edge. 'I assume you're leaving?'

His question had tears pricking her eyes.

She knew that Richard had been up all night working, and it sounded as if he'd had the most dreadful day. Sorcha knew she was a good nurse—but possibly not the best support to have at times like this...

'I can get a refund...' She sniffed. 'Richard, can we talk?'

'Yes.'

'I've got so many questions.'

'I know you have.'

'I'll wait here at the station.'

'Thanks,' he said, and rang off.

He watched the night close in as the train approached London.

And when he eventually arrived at Kings Cross, he saw her straight away, with that mane of hair he'd recognise anywhere.

She was sitting at the café where they'd passed all those hours away, and she'd been crying.

Sorcha didn't do tears very often, and had splashed her face with water and even put on some concealer.

Then she saw him.

He had on his big grey coat and black jeans, and somehow, even after being up for more than twenty-four hours, he still looked suave. Her heart soared when she saw him.

'Hey.'

He didn't play games, or sulk. Instead he gave her a kiss on the cheek and took a seat.

'I overreacted,' she said.

'You're pregnant, in a different country, with a guy who—'

'I adore,' Sorcha told him. 'But...'

'Say it.'

'I can't...'

'You can.'

She shook her head.

'I am sorry I couldn't let you know what was happening,' he said. 'I'd finished work, done a bit of shopping... I was just coming into the Underground when Trefor called. I was talking to him and Jess's doctor on the train when my phone died.'

'What happened to Jess?'

'Seizures,' Richard said. 'Prolonged.'

'I kept telling myself that something must have come up...that maybe you'd been late leaving work, or Jess... I just didn't understand why you couldn't call.'

'Sorcha,' he said. 'Next time—and there will undoubtedly be a next time—instead of trying to work out why, tell yourself that I love you and that there must be a good reason.'

She started when he said that, and her eyes shot up to warn him. 'Please don't just say that.'

'I do love you, though.' He stared at her with

those gorgeous blue eyes. 'I would never say it unless I was certain, and I wasn't certain until today…but I love you.'

She swallowed. 'What happened this morning?'

'I just knew…' he said. 'I know you've been through a lot, and I know things are very up and down in my life. I had to be sure.'

'So all those times we made love you didn't know…?' She stopped, but only because he'd smiled.

'I thought I might…then I was sure I did…' Then perhaps he saw her frown. 'I've been in love,' he said. 'I thought I knew what it was. I didn't realise it could be so different.'

'We're different.'

'Not just that…' He shook his head. 'I didn't believe people who said they fell in love in a matter of days. It doesn't make sense to me. Or it didn't. But I think we fell in love that first night. I just took a few weeks to realise it.'

'A lot of weeks!'

'Sorcha, I dated Jess for seven years, I was engaged to her for five…'

He didn't want to compare, but he was finding out that was the bewildering beauty of love, and he chose to try to explain it.

'Falling in love with Jess was like…climbing

a mountain together.' He watched Sorcha's lips pinch in jealousy. 'Falling in love with you was like bungee jumping.'

She actually laughed.

'Or diving off a cliff.'

'You really love me?'

'Yes—and it feels selfish. I'm not in a position to marry you… I can't promise my phone won't go and I'll have to rush off again…' He leant forward and took her hands. 'I *can* promise you that I'd do the same for you.'

'You already have,' Sorcha said. 'On Christmas Day.'

'Yes.' He smiled. 'You had questions…?'

He looked at her eyes, felt them scanning his, and even with all the questions she must have he could see the deep well of understanding waiting to emerge, and he gave her time for it.

She took in a shaky breath.

'Ask anything…' he invited, as he always had.

'I'm scared you'll feel stuck with me.'

'Like you think your parents feel?' He was possibly being too direct, but it had to be said. 'Because I happen to disagree. I think they love you. A lot.'

'You haven't even met them.'

'I've heard you talking to them, and it sounds like a pretty great relationship. And they came to Manchester that time…' He looked at her. 'I think they're worried about Amanda hurting you. I know I am.'

'I'm not just talking about my parents.'

'About Jess?' he asked. 'No.' He shook his head. 'I never thought I'd come close to feeling happy again, but I am. And if you knew how I felt when I met you, you'd know how deep the love I have for you is.'

'I know how much you love her…'

He nodded.

'And I keep thinking…' She clearly didn't know how to describe it. 'What if we'd met when Jess was okay?'

He frowned.

'If Jess had been at the conference and that thing with Edward had happened…' She swallowed. 'What would have happened to us?'

'Nothing.'

She stared back. 'I feel guilty,' she admitted.

'Please don't.'

'I still remember how dreadful I felt that morning, thinking that I could have broken up a marriage.'

'Not mine,' he said. 'Sorcha, you're not the first beautiful woman I've seen, and I'm not going to pretend like some guys that I don't even notice, but nothing would have happened between us.'

'You sound very sure.'

'Because I am sure,' he told her. 'I'll tell you

exactly what would have happened. I'd have taken you to this table, bought you some drinks and snacks and made sure you were okay, and then I'd have gone.'

She nodded. 'Would you move to Scotland if I asked you?' she asked.

'I'd hoped you wouldn't ask me that again.'

'I'm asking if you would.'

And he looked right into her green eyes and knew she was challenging him, and he didn't blame her one bit. He was asking her to give up her life there because of his own chaotic life.

'No.'

He watched the column of her throat as she swallowed and knew that might have sounded harsh, especially as she was pregnant with his child, but it had been written on his heart long ago.

'The only way I can explain it,' he said, 'is to say that if the same thing happened to you—God forbid—I wouldn't move a ten-hour journey away.'

And it might be the wrong answer for some, but for Sorcha it was perfect.

'Sorcha, if you do need to be close to your family then I'll make it work… I'll commute, and then later…'

His voice husked, and she knew what that difficult pause meant.

'When it's just us, then I'll move up to Scotland...'

When he gave his love it really was for ever.

Not just in good times, but right to the end, and for someone who had been so badly let down from the cradle it meant the world.

'Come on,' he said, and stood.

She thought they were heading for the Underground, but he led them out of the station.

'Where are we going?'

'Guess...'

It was the hotel where they'd gone that first night, and where they'd welcomed in the New Year.

'Why are we here?'

'Because I want you. And the Tube would take too long to get us home,' he said, carrying her holdall as they walked through the crisp winter night.

The foyer was almost empty, and there was no one jumping out on them at the lifts—just dark and quiet and tranquillity.

'Sorry about this,' he said, picking up his phone as they stepped into the lift. 'I've got a lot of people asking after Jess. I'll just send a message.'

She watched as he put his day into a few lines.

'What are people going to say about us?' she asked.

'I think most of my friendship group knows. I've been getting a lot of messages asking how I am.'

'What about your family?'

'Gemma knows.'

'Jess's family?'

'I told Trefor today.'

'How was he?'

'He'll get there,' Richard said assuredly. 'I know he will.'

She looked over at him and thought she had never known someone as strong and yet as kind as him.

He swiped the keycard in the door of their hotel room and she saw the fairies had been in—a different lot.

There were candles in hurricane glasses, a silver tray with chocolate truffles and flowers, and an ice bucket filled with bottles of sparkling water.

'I didn't really bring you here to ravish you…' he started.

'That's not fair,' Sorcha said, and she put her arms around his neck and kissed his tired mouth.

He shrugged off his coat, and then there were her boots and scarves. He unwrapped her like a parcel and kissed her down onto the bed.

They didn't even get in it.

They rolled together, kissing and turning, finding the tender places they needed to be, their legs scissoring each other's, taking their time to explore the other.

'Lucky me,' Sorcha said—because that was how he made her feel every day.

It was a delicious climax, watching each other, driving each other to the edge, and then just lying locked together afterwards.

Richard was on his back and Sorcha on her side, one leg over him and her coconut scented hair tickling his face. He smoothed it away.

'Stay still,' Richard said, and she frowned. 'I just felt the baby move…'

Just this little nudge…and he really wasn't imagining things.

He rolled her onto her back and, yes, their baby was moving. He felt the little kicks, and asked again about the scan.

'It was incredible,' she said. 'They're going to send us the films.'

'I can't wait,' he said, and frowned as Sorcha rolled off the bed.

Even if she was the most comfortable she'd ever been, she did have a surprise for him.

She went to her bag.

"I've got something for you…'

She pulled out the image and handed it to him.

'Meet your son.'
'You found out?'
'I did.'
'He's beautiful…'

And she knew that wasn't just a proud father speaking. It was the most incredibly detailed image…tiny nails and beautiful lips.

He stared at the image for a very long time, looking as entranced as she had been.

'I'm sorry I wasn't there.'

He wasn't so much apologising, but he was sorry to have missed it, she knew.

'I know,' Sorcha said. 'Next time.'

'Yes…'

He put the image down.

'Sorcha, you've ruined my plans.'

'I know. Nappies all the way now.'

'No, I meant for tonight. I booked the room this morning.'

'I thought it was a last-minute thing?'

'No.'

It was Richard's turn to roll from the bed and she watched as he reached into his coat.

'This morning, before it all kicked off, I went to the jeweller's where I got your watch…' He pulled out a box, and though it was her third box in only a few months, this one was little, and velvet, and if she hadn't known his circumstances she might have thought he was about to propose.

'What is it?' she asked.

'Open it and see.'

Perhaps he saw her nerves. 'It's not an engagement ring, Sorcha,' he said. 'We'll do all that when the time is right.'

Earrings, she decided, and vowed to love them even before she'd prised open the velvet lid.

She gasped when she saw a ring, and its glittering diamonds. He took it from the box. It was a semi-circle of diamonds, in silver or platinum—whatever metal it was, Sorcha didn't care. It was simply the ring she needed from him…

'It's an eternity ring,' Richard said.

'Yes…' She watched it blurring through her tears.

'I chose it because it means for ever. And, yes, it's unconventional to start with that, but…' He looked at her and she knew he told her a truth. 'I want yours to be the last face I see…'

They were the words she'd used on the day they'd met.

'It's beautiful…'

She looked up to the eyes that always steadied her. It was in the gaps, the times in between, when he wasn't there that the old fears surfaced, the constant terror of being left. But moored in his gaze she felt safe.

His love was a gift.

This really was a for ever love.

'Tomorrow,' he told her, 'I'm going to introduce myself to your parents, and we're going to tell them about the baby together.'

It was a blissful night, and in the morning they took the train to her home.

In a few hours they'd be official.

Well, they already were.

But for a moment it was still a lovely secret, waiting to be shared.

'Have you told them we're coming?' he asked.

'I have,' Sorcha said, and she could not stop smiling.

As the train pulled into Waverly she saw the castle, proud and looming, and she felt the gorgeous sense of being overwhelmed it delivered every time...

'Heart squeezing?' he checked.

'Always.'

'Let's go and meet your family.'

EPILOGUE

EXAM DAY DAWNED.

And it was a day that had been missed or cancelled too many times.

That would not be happening today.

Richard came out of the shower on a puff of steam and started to get dressed, but his eyes were watching her, as if he knew she was not being completely honest with him.

'Sorcha…?'

'Mm…?' she responded, taking a sip of tea, pretending she didn't know what he was asking as he clipped on his watch.

'Is everything okay?'

'Of course it is.'

Sorcha refused to be in early labour.

She wasn't having contractions—just a little tightening now and then. Braxton Hicks, she was completely sure. But she knew if he got even a hint, he wouldn't leave.

He came over and sat on the bed, put a hand on her stomach.

'What are you doing?' she asked, all affronted.

'You're acting strange.'

'I am not,' she said, and put the mug down. 'I'm nervous for you.'

She put her hand up and felt his gorgeous smooth jaw, then wiped a tiny bit of shaving cream from his ear and willed her uterus to behave.

'He's awake,' Richard said, as they both watched the performing circus that was her stomach.

'Very,' Sorcha said. 'Richard, you really do need to go.'

He nodded, and removed his hand from her stomach. He gave her a light kiss goodbye, but then lingered in her embrace.

'Good luck,' she said.

He pulled away and then stood. 'You'll call me if anything changes?'

The flat felt very silent after he'd gone, and she lay down for a while, relieved she hadn't told him, because really nothing was happening.

For once the gorgeous view of London didn't distract her, even on a bright blue May day, and she found she kept checking the time. At eleven, when she knew the first exam would have started, she wandered into his study.

She picked up a heavy paperweight and then replaced it, then turned and looked at the photo of Richard and Jess. There were several of Sorcha and he around the apartment, but his wedding photo was here, not prominent, or looming over their bed or anything awkward…

Jess had died in March, with her husband and loving family around her and her closest friends…

All as it should have been.

Sorcha had gone home for a few days rather than sit alone in the apartment, and she'd spent some time with her mum…found out a few things.

Her mum had cried when she'd found out she was pregnant with Theresa. 'You were such a cheeky wee baby…we just didn't know how we'd manage…'

Her own baby was being a bit cheeky…

She took a deep breath and felt the hard rock of her stomach.

That wasn't a Braxton Hicks.

Oh, God…

She went to call Richard…to tell him that, actually, he ought to get here. But then she looked at the time. The second exam would be starting…

First labours last for ages, she told herself, and checked her book.

She lay on the bed, but then another pain came, and so she started to time them.

She rang the midwife.

'They're quite irregular,' she told her, but no, her waters hadn't broken.

And then they did—just as she was on the phone to her mum.

Her mother was a little dramatic with her advice, she thought—to Sorcha, it was almost a code violation for an A&E nurse to call an ambulance for herself. You had to be actually dying or…

Giving birth.

'I think it's coming,' Sorcha told the controller. 'I might be wrong…'

She went back to the view, resting her head on her forearm, just too deep inside herself to think of answering the ringing phone. She stared at the streets and the stations and knew that somewhere out there Richard was making his way home.

Relief rushed over her when she heard the elevator, then the thud of footsteps.

'Hello?' She heard a female voice. 'Ambulance—where are you?'

'Through here.'

She looked up, then did a double-take—because walking behind the lady was an oddly familiar face.

'I know you…' he said.

'Luke!'

It was the paramedic from that day at the hospital.

'How are you, Sorcha?' he asked, then told his partner how they knew each other.

'Richard has exams today. I'm scared he's going to miss the birth.'

'How far away is he?'

'An hour or so?'

She wasn't certain—but she rather thought she saw Luke and his partner share a small smile.

'I think,' the treating paramedic said, 'that he has every chance of making it. Do you think you can walk to the elevator?'

'Walk?' Sorcha gave an incredulous snort.

Richard made it in plenty of time!

'You knew,' he scolded, taking her in his arms.

'I didn't.'

She swallowed and just breathed him in, simply relieved he was here.

'I had the tiniest twinges... Nothing really happened until you were on your way home. Football players have to do it,' she said. 'They have to play in the final and things...'

The midwife nodded. 'And the military.'

'I'm not a footballer—nor in the military.'

It was a very quiet birth.

Sorcha went right into herself and pushed life into the world, and Richard was there, kind and constant.

And he was so calm that even Sorcha, who knew him better than anyone else on the planet, saw nothing in the glance he shared with the midwife as she checked the baby's heartrate.

'I can't do this…' she said at last, shaking her head. 'It's been hours.'

'It's not much longer now,' he said.

'You keep saying that!'

'Sorcha…'

She looked up in surprise to see Monica, tying on an apron as she read the CTG.

'Is everything okay?' she asked.

'Baby's not liking the contractions,' Monica explained. 'So when the next one comes I want you to really push.'

'I already am!'

'I know you've been working hard, but when the next contraction comes you're going to push for England, Sorcha. Got it?'

'I'm Scottish,' Sorcha snapped, masking a slight panic that something was going wrong, but Monica seemed unfazed, the midwife too, and Richard was his usual measured self.

She felt that certain feeling of calm that always descended when she met his gaze.

Confident.

Safe.

He wouldn't let her fall.

'You've got this,' he told her, and that took away her fear. And somehow she was free to do what she had to.

She pushed for more than Scotland or England. It felt as if she was pushing out an entire globe.

'Save your breath,' Monica warned when she shouted out. 'One more push.'

And then he was here.

Sorcha glimpsed big eyes and brown hair, and a very affronted look... He was long and tall and delivered high onto her tummy, and she pulled him to her chest, where he shivered and let out a husky cry.

A blanket was placed over him and she saw Richard's finger stroking his cheek. Then his hand was pulled away, and she looked up and saw his fingers were pressed into his eyes.

She'd never seen him cry.

Oh, Sorcha had guessed a couple of times that of course he must have, but now she saw this beautiful man surrender to emotion for a moment. And when she touched his cheek he gripped her hand. Today he didn't cry alone.

Life was precious...every second of it—even the storms that swept you away only to bring you back in.

'He's a mini you,' Sorcha said, already utterly in love, stroking her baby's straight brown hair and watching it fall into perfect shape. 'He looks like he's just been to the barber's.'

'Look at those eyes,' he said as they opened—they were almond-shaped, like Sorcha's. 'They're yours.'

'They *are* mine...' She nodded, fascinated to see a part of herself in her child.

'Baby Lewis,' the midwife announced. 'Born at five minutes past twelve.'

Sorcha looked up at the clock and saw that it was just after midnight.

And that felt right.

It really was a brand-new day.

'Do you have a name?' the midwife asked.

'James,' Sorcha said, because it was her dad's name—her real dad...the one who had raised her.

Or perhaps because it was the only name they'd been able to agree on.

'Nice and conservative,' Richard had pointed out.

And Sorcha was more than content with that.

* * * * *

*If you enjoyed this story,
check out these other great reads
from Carol Marinelli*

One Month to Tame the Surgeon
The Nurse's Pregnancy Wish
Unlocking the Doctor's Secrets
The Nurse's Reunion Wish

All available now!

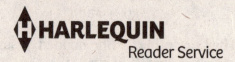

Enjoyed your book?

Try the perfect subscription for Romance readers and get more great books like this delivered right to your door.

See why over 10+ million readers have tried Harlequin Reader Service.

Start with a Free Welcome Collection with free books and a gift—valued over $20.

Choose any series in print or ebook.
See website for details and order today:

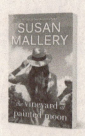 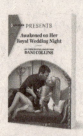 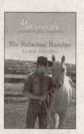 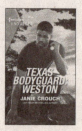

TryReaderService.com/subscriptions